TINNITUS
TREATMENT TOOLBOX

TINNITUS TREATMENT TOOLBOX

A Guide for People with Ear Noise

J. L. Mayes

Order this book online at www.trafford.com
or email orders@trafford.com

Most Trafford titles are also available at major online book retailers.

Printed in the United States of America.

ISBN: 978-1-4269-1215-3 (sc)
ISBN: 978-1-4269-1216-0 (hc)
ISBN: 978-1-4269-1217-7 (e)

Library of Congress Control Number: 2012915124

Trafford rev. December 06, 2012

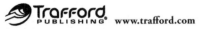 www.trafford.com

North America & international
toll-free: 1 888 232 4444 (USA & Canada)
phone: 250 383 6864 ♦ fax: 812 355 4082

I would like to thank Bud and Pauline Wilkinson who made it possible for me to become an audiologist, as well as everyone who has given me encouragement, support or helpful feedback while writing this book: Sharon Adelman, Sandra Aristizabal, Kristina Bingham, Dr. Nirvana Kiarostami, Carol Lau, Murray Leslie, Clarissa Mayes, Samantha Mayes, Marilyn Miller, Jeanne Moskalyk, Kukuh Noertjojo, Glynnis Tidball, Dr. Anna Van Maanen, Dennis Wilkinson, and most importantly of all Diane Wilkinson and Brad Mayes.

This book is dedicated:
To my husband for his unwavering love and support.
To my daughters for my joy and inspiration.
To my family for their devotion.
To my colleagues for their wisdom and dedication.
To my clients for their courage, humour, and perseverance.

CONTENTS

INTRODUCTION

Through knowledge, creating health. University of British Columbia. Faculty of Medicine Vision Statement.

Tinnitus is a name given to noises in the ears that people hear when there is no outside noise source. In other words, you are hearing something that nobody else can hear. It is extremely common. Why don't people talk about it? It is probably because tinnitus is also invisible to other people's eyes and ears. People with tinnitus often feel uncomfortable telling other people "I hear noises in my ears (or head), but nobody else can hear them." As an audiologist doing hearing tests and counselling, I have often been the first person people have told about their tinnitus. I have also personally had tinnitus for over 20 years, and telling people about it has never come up naturally in conversation. Tinnitus is very much a hidden symptom.

Tinnitus is commonly pronounced [tin-it-us] or [tin-night-us]. Both pronunciations are fine. Tinnitus can be described as different sound types (or combinations of sounds) including ring, roar, hiss, screech, whistle, buzz, click, hum, etc. Tinnitus comes from the Latin and means "jingling ear". Usually only the person with the tinnitus hears it. Tinnitus is not an imaginary sound. Tinnitus may be in one ear, both ears, or in the head. It may be there constantly or occasionally. It may be any loudness from soft to loud. Typically it changes from time to time. There is a rumor that Vincent Van Gogh may have cut off his ear in an attempt to get rid of tinnitus.

Tinnitus is not a disease, illness or disorder. As this book will explain, tinnitus is naturally produced by the hearing system. Tinnitus may be temporary or permanent (chronic). There are simple and effective approaches available to help people overcome any distress they experience from this harmless sound. In case there is a medical cause, it is always recommended you get the approval of your doctor and/or ear specialist before you begin a tinnitus treatment plan. The presence of the following conditions always requires medical attention. See your doctor if you have:

- Newly started tinnitus.
- Tinnitus in one ear only.
- Pulse-like tinnitus.
- Tinnitus that sounds like voices.
- Sudden or rapidly worsening tinnitus.
- Better hearing in one ear than the other.
- Dizziness (vertigo) or imbalance.
- Sudden or rapidly worsening hearing loss in one or both ears.
- Drainage, pain or discomfort in one or both ears.
- Anxiety, depression or suicidal thoughts.

In many cases, there is no specific medical condition found as the tinnitus cause. This is why tinnitus is often described as idiopathic or cause unknown. After finding out there is no medical treatment needed, many people experience increased tinnitus distress after being told to "just learn to live with it" without any practical "how to" recommendations. Whether there is an underlying medical condition to your tinnitus or not, the same non-medical tinnitus treatment approaches work. I know that people with tinnitus can significantly improve their sense of well-being through treatment tools.

I wrote this book to help share the message that there are many treatment options available that can greatly help people with tinnitus distress. Successful coping is a realistic goal. People get the most benefit from a tinnitus treatment program customized for their individual needs. The tinnitus care provider(s) involved will depend on the treatment needed. Treatment takes time. It takes time to incorporate changes (treatment strategies) into your daily life. It takes time to see results. The longer you have had tinnitus, the longer it typically takes to notice change. Tinnitus is a complex condition. A simplistic approach is not realistic. You will likely need to make changes for your ears, mind and body to maximize success.

This book does not give a quick fix or a cure. It does give an overview of available treatments to help you become familiar with the tools to consider for your personal tinnitus treatment toolbox. Try the tools that speak directly to your individual needs, and keep using the ones that are helpful or beneficial. These approaches are typically most effective when the person with tinnitus has the support and guidance of a sympathetic and knowledgeable care provider. This book can't replace specific medical or tinnitus treatment advice from your care provider(s). Only they can answer questions specific to you, and help make sure the choice of care is appropriate.

Author's Case: In 1986, I suffered whiplash and concussion in a motor vehicle accident. While most of my injuries healed over time, I was left with a loud buzzing in my ears called tinnitus. I repeatedly went to doctors and ear specialists asking why I now had this noise and what I could do about it. I was told it was nothing and I should just learn to live with it. Because of my interest in tinnitus, I became an audiologist. It was disappointing to discover that there was little to offer at that time to people suffering from bothersome tinnitus.

My tinnitus grew worse. It was a non-stop buzz, overriding other noises and voices around me. Sometimes it would escalate for a minute or two to a piercing shriek before settling back down. At these times I would panic. If it stayed like that, I would never be able to stand it. I decided quiet was the answer. I fought with my husband over the radio and TV volume. I stayed away from groups of people or "noisy" places like malls or restaurants.

Life became restricted. Due to other medical reasons involving chronic pain and fatigue, I went on disability leave. Despite spending several months in the quiet of my home, there was no improvement in my tinnitus. I read of various potential triggers and began to keep a detailed diary, searching for some change I could make in diet or routine that might lead to a cure. My tinnitus became even worse. Over a decade passed of listening to non-stop tinnitus from the moment I woke in the morning until I tried to fall asleep at night. I thought that nothing could ever help.

Then scientific research began appearing which described new treatment approaches for people with bothersome tinnitus. I discovered that my preference for silence and my habit of daily monitoring of my tinnitus was very counter-productive. Researchers also began to discuss the similarities between chronic tinnitus and chronic pain. I took treatment information from the scientific literature on tinnitus, pain, and alternative healing. Using this as a basis, I created a personal tinnitus treatment plan for myself.

After many months, I experienced a significant decrease in my tinnitus. I have continued to try promising new treatment approaches that over time have greatly improved my ability to cope with my tinnitus. I tried a variety of different tools that spoke directly to my needs, and over time found which ones worked best for me. I ended up with a smaller number of tools that were effective for my tinnitus. Some tools I use daily. Other tools I use as needed.

I am now rarely aware of my tinnitus. When I do think of it, the intensity and pitch are usually a soft to medium hiss. This is much easier to cope with than the longstanding constant screeching I had heard for years before starting my tinnitus treatment plan. My tinnitus still flares up sometimes. But I know which tools work for me. I can dip into my tinnitus treatment toolbox to make the flare-ups shorter and less severe. I believe anyone with tinnitus can also put together his or her own individual tinnitus treatment toolbox to live without distress and cope well regardless of tinnitus.

HOW WE HEAR

Music is the arithmetic of sounds. Claude Debussy.

In order to better understand tinnitus, it is helpful to understand the normal hearing system. A very basic description is given here only as background information to help understand how the hearing system is involved with tinnitus. The hearing or auditory system is highly specialized for sound processing. Sound travels in waves. If you drop a pebble in a pool of water, it will create ripples that travel out from where the pebble fell in. Similarly sound waves travel through air, rippling out from their sound source. Our hearing system processes incoming sound waves. The brain uses this information to perceive and interpret the sounds in our environment (e.g. voices, nature, music, machines, etc.).

There are two main features of sound waves: pitch (frequency) and loudness (intensity). The pitch or frequency of a sound depends on how many sound waves reach the ear in a given period of time. For example, when sound waves move slowly then fewer reach the ear in a given period of time. This results in a lower pitch or a deeper sound (e.g. a foghorn). When sound waves move quickly, then more reach the ear in a given period of time. This results in a higher pitch or squeakier sound (e.g. a bird chirping). Sound frequency is measured in Hertz (Hz). The normal frequency range of human hearing is 20 to 20,000 Hz. However, the range from 250 to 8000 Hz is considered most important for speech communication.

The loudness or intensity of a sound depends on how large the sound waves are that reach the ear. For example, the larger the sound waves the louder the sound (e.g. a shout). The smaller the sound waves the softer the sound (e.g. a whisper). Sound intensity or sound power is measured in decibels (dB). The normal loudness range of human hearing sensitivity is 0 dB to 140 dB. This range covers soft whispers to painfully loud sounds. In general a 3 dB increase is equivalent to doubling the loudness (e.g. 23 dB is approximately twice as loud as 20 dB). The value of 0 dB is not silence. It is the softest sound a normal hearing young adult can detect. Sound intensities of 85 dB or higher have the potential to damage the hearing system depending on how long you listen to the sound.

SOUND CONDUCTION (OUTER AND MIDDLE EAR)

Sounds waves travel through two main sections of the hearing system: the ears (peripheral) and the brain (central). The system starts with sound conduction through the ears or peripheral section. The ears are actually divided into three main anatomical parts: the outer, middle and inner ear. Sounds waves traveling in air around a listener's head enter through the outer ear. The outer ear starts with the visible part of the ear on the sides of our heads that is technically called the "pinna". This is the part of the ear often used to hang earrings or glasses on. The pinna acts as a funnel that collects sound waves and directs them down the ear canal. The ear canal is typically considered part of the outer ear. The outer section of the ear canal is where hair and earwax is produced. The ear canal is designed to help protect the eardrum from incoming debris (e.g. dirt, bugs, etc.).

The middle ear starts at the eardrum that sits at the end of the ear canal. Behind the eardrum, there are three tiny interconnected middle ear bones: the hammer, anvil and stirrup (the malleus, incus and stapes respectively). The middle ear bones sit in an air filled space between the eardrum and the inner ear. This space is ventilated by the Eustachian tube. The Eustachian tube leads from the middle ear space to the back of the throat. It keeps the pressure equal between the middle ear space and the outside atmosphere. Usually this tube stays closed, and only opens briefly during yawning or swallowing. If the Eustachian tube stops opening properly because of infection, allergies or other conditions (e.g. rapidly landing in an airplane), it can cause a feeling of fullness or pain in the ears. Some people notice a slight popping or crackling sound when their Eustachian tube(s) open and close. During large yawns, temporary changes in tinnitus characteristics can also occur (e.g. increased loudness).

The middle ear turns sound waves traveling from the outer ear into a mechanical vibration. The eardrum vibrates to incoming sound waves similar to the cone of a loudspeaker. This vibratory energy flows through the middle ear bones, which deliver the sound energy to the inner ear fluids in a piston like action. An important complex function of the middle ear system is to change sound wave energy from air transmission (outer and middle ear pathway) into fluid transmission once it reaches the inner ear pathway. Without the middle ear, sound waves in air would simply reflect off the inner ear fluids leading to a large loss of sound energy. A working middle ear system effectively transfers sound energy through to the inner ear.

When a hearing loss is from a problem with how sound is carried through the outer and/or middle ear pathways, the hearing loss is called "conductive". This type of hearing loss can make speech or other sounds appear muffled or soft. Hearing loss from the outer ear(s) is often temporary although more longstanding conditions can occur. This type of hearing loss is often related to outer ear infections or too much earwax (cerumen). When people have problems with their middle ear(s), significant hearing loss can be present. Middle ear problems are most commonly related to infection but causes can also include trauma, head injury, and Otosclerosis (hereditary middle ear bone changes). The amount of hearing loss depends on which part of the middle ear is affected (eardrum and/or middle ear bones) and whether the problem is temporary or longstanding. Conductive hearing loss can often be corrected by medical treatment (medicine or surgery). Sometimes hearing aids are also needed. Tinnitus is common in people with conductive hearing loss.

Case 1: He could not clear his ears on an airplane when coming home from vacation. He experienced tinnitus and severe ear pain in his left ear after landing. Testing showed that his eardrum had burst. An ear infection started, and medication was prescribed. He had a conductive hearing loss. The eardrum healed over. The tinnitus faded away over time. The hearing returned to normal.

Case 2: Her ear infections started in childhood. She still gets occasional infections as an adult. She has had several ear surgeries including placement of tubes in the eardrums. She has scarred eardrums and stiff middle ear bone movement. She has a permanent conductive hearing loss that is worse when she has an ear infection. She hears tinnitus regularly, but it gets louder during an infection.

Case 3: He fell off a ladder and landed on his head. He suffered a severe concussion, tinnitus and hearing loss. Testing showed the force of the blow had dislocated the middle ear bones in his right ear. This caused a conductive hearing loss. Surgery was done to help fix the middle ear bones. He still has slightly uneven hearing between his ears. His tinnitus has become less noticeable over time.

Case 4: She began to notice hearing loss and tinnitus after her second child was born. Hearing testing and medical referral led to a diagnosis of Otosclerosis. Otosclerosis is a bony growth on the middle ear bones that stops them from moving properly. Treatment included surgery and hearing aids.

SOUND INPUT (INNER EAR)

The inner ear is made up of a hearing system and a balance system (that will not be described here). When the inner ear is discussed in this book, it is only referring to the hearing system. The inner ear is a small snail shaped bony structure called the cochlea. It is well supplied by blood vessels and nerves. The cochlea has an extremely complicated structure and mechanism that will not be described in detail here. Simply, the cochlea is filled with fluid, and contains thousands of tiny microscopic hair cells. The cochlea receives sound vibrations from the middle ear that stimulate these hair cells. There are approximately 15,000 hair cells per ear. These hair cells respond to the pitch and loudness of incoming sound waves and change the sound vibrations into electrical impulses.

Once sound vibrations are changed into electrical impulses at the inner ear, a message is sent to the brain signaling the presence of sound and providing detailed information about it. At this point, all sounds from the outside environment are mixed together. These electrical impulses are carried up nerve fibers in the auditory or hearing nerve through to the brain where information is processed.

The normal sound pathway to the cochlea is called "air conduction". However, if the whole skull is set into vibration (e.g. from an extremely intense sound or through contact with vibration), sound energy can be delivered to the cochlea without traveling down the normal middle ear pathway. This type of sound simulation to the inner ear is called "bone conduction". Both air conduction and bone conduction stimuli may be used during hearing testing in order to locate problems within the hearing system. Air conduction testing checks the status of the middle and inner ears in combination. Bone conduction testing checks the status of the inner ear alone.

Hearing loss from problems in the inner ear or auditory nerve is called "sensorineural". This type of hearing problem can't be detected by a physical examination since the outer ear and eardrum will look normal. This type of hearing loss makes it difficult to understand speech, especially when there is background noise present. There are multiple causes of sensorineural hearing loss including aging, heredity, hazardous noise, viral infections, cardiovascular disease, drugs toxic to the ears, etc. Sensorineural hearing loss is permanent. There is no medicine or surgery to correct this type of hearing loss. Hearing aids are the standard treatment. When sensorineural and conductive hearing loss components are both present, the hearing loss is called "mixed". This type of hearing loss can only improve as much as the conductive component can be corrected. Tinnitus is common in people with sensorineural or mixed hearing loss.

Case 5: This 62 year old noticed difficulties hearing at the coffee shop for several years. She also began to have problems hearing on the telephone, and her family complained the TV was too loud. She also noticed tinnitus that had started gradually. Testing showed sensorineural hearing loss that appeared to be age-related.

Case 6: This 57 year old had worked in the construction industry for 20 years. In the early days, no hearing protection was provided. Now he used earmuffs. He noticed tinnitus that had been there for a long time. He thought the tinnitus was interfering with conversations. Testing showed a sensorineural hearing loss that was likely related to working in hazardous noise.

Case 7: She began to have episodes of swirling dizziness. During these episodes she noticed ear fullness, tinnitus and poorer hearing. Over a period of years, testing showed fluctuating sensorineural hearing loss. Her ear specialist diagnosed Meniere's disease.

Case 8: He was chopping down a tree when a large branch fell on his head. He was unconscious for several hours. At the hospital, tests showed a skull fracture that ran through his left inner ear. After this accident, he reported problems hearing and loud tinnitus in his left ear. Testing showed a left ear sensorineural hearing loss.

Case 9: He was born with significant sensorineural hearing loss. One morning he woke up to discover a sudden worsening of his hearing loss in his right ear along with a buzzing sound. He saw his doctor immediately. Medical examination showed his right ear canal was completely blocked by earwax. A temporary mixed hearing loss (conductive and sensorineural) was present. The conductive hearing loss and tinnitus cleared up after the doctor removed the earwax. This left the permanent sensorineural loss.

Case 10: She noticed sudden hearing loss in her left ear along with ringing and dizziness. She immediately went to the emergency department at her local hospital, and saw an ear specialist. An inner ear viral infection was suspected. Medical treatment including medication was started as soon as possible. Although her hearing partly returned, she still had a permanent sensorineural hearing loss and tinnitus.

SOUND PROCESSING (THE BRAIN)

The outer, middle and inner ears are primarily the sound pick-up mechanism. After traveling through the peripheral system and then along the hearing or auditory nerve, the sound pathway changes to a series of nerve fiber networks within the brain. There are approximately 30,000 nerve fibers in the hearing nerve that lead into approximately 10 million fibers in the brain's hearing system networks. It is these nerve fiber networks that are responsible for perception of sound. We hear with our brain. The hearing system in the brain is always in a state of readiness. Nerve fibers are never completely quiet. Like a car in neutral, there is always a certain amount of background activity going on. When system activity increases like an accelerating engine, then further processing happens to determine if the activity is important or not.

The brain interprets these patterns of increased nerve fiber activity as our sound environment. All sounds (e.g. a dog barking, a voice, raindrops, birdsong) will have their own unique pattern inside the hearing system. When nerve fiber activity matching known patterns comes through the hearing system, then it is heard as the corresponding sound. Different patterns of nerve fiber activity happen for silence. Our hearing system is designed to let us hear sound as well as no sound. Many nerve fibers actually become more active for decreased or softer sound input. Lower sound input can come from a quiet or silent environment. Sound input can also be lower when a person develops hearing loss. When less sound input comes through the peripheral hearing system (outer, middle and inner ears), this will cause more activity from the nerve fibers tuned for this. Silence or soft sounds in the environment can signal danger for humans. A snapping twig in a forest can mean a bear is hunting nearby. A creaking floorboard can mean a thief is in a house. A hearing system designed to process a range of soft to loud sounds as well as process silence is essential for human safety.

Day and night, our hearing systems continually process a constant stream of information about our sound environment. The initial work of the hearing system takes place without us even being aware it is going on. It happens completely subconsciously. The hearing system screens incoming activity and delivers only the most important signals through the system. Imagine the hearing system works like an elevator stopping at each floor in a tall building. The basement may be full of potential information about our sound environment. But as information flows up the elevator, nerve fibers at each floor are working to check for patterns. If patterns are identified as unimportant, the information is filtered out. This information does not make it to the next floor. If patterns are recognized as potentially important, this information does make it to higher levels as the nerve fibers continue trying to check the pattern.

Once past the subconscious networks, the higher levels of the hearing system in the brain analyze nerve fiber patterns further. More areas of the brain like those needed for language can also become active. At this point, a person finally becomes consciously aware of their sound environment. Processing at this level includes identifying that a sound is heard, recognizing what the sound is (e.g. a car horn, music, speech), and interpreting the sound if necessary (e.g. understanding what was said).

Although either ear alone can do most sound processing, the second ear is not a backup system in case something happens to the other ear. Both ears need to work together for several very important parts of sound processing. This includes ability to locate or find a sound source (e.g. where did a sound come from) and for selective listening (e.g. listening to one sound or voice while screening out background sounds).

Table 1

HOW SOUND IS HEARD

1.	Sound from environment moves through ear system.	**Sound In**
2.	Nerve fiber activity starts and sound message is carried through brain.	**Sound Processing**
3.	Sound is heard.	

HOW WE HEAR TINNITUS

What shall possess them with the heaviest sound that ever yet they heard? William Shakespeare (Macbeth).

TINNITUS EXISTENCE

There is an old philosophical question that asks: If a tree falls in a forest, does it make a sound? The frequently suggested answer is that it can't make a sound if nobody is there to hear it. The hearing system nerve fiber networks are responsible for all perception of sound. If there was no working hearing system near the tree, then there was no sound. Consider a different question: If no tree falls in a forest, does it make a sound? In the case of people with tinnitus, the answer is yes. Nerve fiber networks in the hearing system can work in such a way that sound is heard even when there was no sound coming from the outside world. People can hear sounds that start from inside the hearing system.

There is a rare type of hearing loss where sound input travels normally through the outer, middle and inner ear, but the brain can't process it. People with this type of hearing loss can't hear sound. If sound travels through the ears but the hearing system in the brain is not working, then no sound is heard. In contrast, the brain often processes information coming from it's own hearing pathways. If the hearing system in the brain becomes active enough, then sound can be heard even when there was no outside sound coming in through the ears. If normal background nerve fiber activity looks like a recognized pattern, then it can easily be sent up the hearing pathways and eventually heard as a sound. It is believed that tinnitus is this type of sound created by our own brain activity.

Research demonstrates that in a quiet enough environment most human beings can hear tinnitus, but it is usually covered up by the variety of noise that floods our environment so that most people aren't aware of it. In 1953, Heller and Bergman did an experiment called *Tinnitus In Normally Hearing Persons*. Everyone had normal hearing and no tinnitus. Each person was placed in a sound proof room for 5 minutes. People were told they were getting a hearing test, but there was actually only 5 minutes of silence. It was found that after 5 minutes, most of the people reported hearing sounds in the head or in their ears identical to those reported by people with tinnitus. This experiment showed that when it is quiet enough, most people could detect the ongoing background activity in the hearing pathways of the brain. This activity is heard as the sound we call tinnitus.

Every living human has this background activity. Some people have suggested that the apparent increase in tinnitus awareness in recent decades may be partly due to modern building technology. Imagine in the Middle Ages a person lives in a drafty castle or hut. The fire is crackling. The straw on the floor crunches as people move around. A person might be far less likely to hear his or her own internal sounds. Consider modern living conditions where people often live and work in well-sealed homes and buildings. Many people try to surround themselves with "peace and quiet". People are far more likely to hear their own internal sounds. However, researchers have found reports of tinnitus dating back to ancient Mesopotamia. It seems tinnitus has actually long been a human condition.

It is not surprising that tinnitus sounds different for different people (e.g. ring, buzz, hiss, beep, whistle). Each of these sounds will have it's own unique pattern in the nerve fiber networks. The brain checks for patterns of activity that match patterns it is already familiar with. Clearly tinnitus is not always generated from the identical nerve fiber patterns in all people otherwise it would sound the same for everybody. With tinnitus, different nerve fibers patterns are likely active for different people. Because the nerve fiber activity is happening within the hearing system, tinnitus is heard as sound. The specific sound will vary from person to person. Tinnitus existence is a human phenomenon. This is only natural. Nobody said our brains work perfectly all the time. Sometimes our hearing systems send an extra "sound message" through our brain. Under the

10

right circumstances (e.g. sufficiently quiet surroundings), anybody can hear it.

Tinnitus existence is likely most commonly seen during a hearing test. Before I test a client's hearing, I ask questions to find out background information (case history) for each new client I see. One of the questions I ask every person is: Do you ever hear any sounds or noises in your ears? Many people say no. Then when I am conducting a hearing test in a sound proof booth, my clients are asked to listen and signal me (raise a hand or press a button) to let me know when they hear even the faintest rings or beeps. This is essentially a repeat of Heller and Bergman's 1953 test conditions except with real sounds. I have worked as an audiologist for many years and tested thousands of people of all ages. The vast majority of people having a hearing test will respond at least once (and for some people many more times) to no sound. They are responding to tinnitus. They are hearing a sound and signal me they have heard something, even though there was no sound delivered to their ear. I see tinnitus existence every day at work. Most often this tinnitus existence is in people who reported no tinnitus when I did my case history interview. Tinnitus simply exists in people. Almost everybody has heard an extra noise in his or her ears every now and then at some time in their life.

Many people also occasionally hear short episodes of beeps or ringing in their ears. This is technically called Transient Spontaneous Tinnitus (TST). Spontaneous tinnitus is a high pitch tinnitus in one or both ears that usually only lasts a few seconds. It often gets louder before fading away. Sometimes the ears feel full or plugged before the spontaneous tinnitus is heard. Spontaneous tinnitus is heard by almost everyone occasionally. People with regular daily tinnitus can still experience spontaneous tinnitus that over-rides their base tinnitus. Typically spontaneous tinnitus for people with chronic tinnitus is louder and may be at a different pitch. Sudden occasional episodes of spontaneous tinnitus can easily make a person fear that their tinnitus will escalate permanently. It is important to remember that spontaneous tinnitus normally occurs in most people and does not signal any permanent change in tinnitus status.

TINNITUS PERSISTENCE

The Heller and Bergman experiment described above raises an important question about tinnitus. The people who entered the experiment with normal healthy ears and no tinnitus also left the experiment with normal healthy ears and no tinnitus. Why didn't the tinnitus last after the people left the sound proof booth? My clients who tell me they have no noises in their ears but respond to tinnitus during their hearing test also walk away without tinnitus. Why does tinnitus persist or last for some people and not for others?

Likely in most people, the brain is able to filter out extra "sound messages" coming from background nerve fiber activity. These messages don't make it past the subconscious nerve fiber networks. However, in some people this extra nerve fiber activity doesn't get screened out. Once this happens, the extra nerve fiber activity could make it through the hearing system on a regular basis. The over activity would typically come from a specific nerve fiber network, so a person's particular tinnitus sound is established (e.g. ring, hiss, buzz). The brain continues to recognize the tinnitus nerve fiber activity as a pattern that should be processed as sound.

In the past, researchers thought that damage to the peripheral hearing system, in particular the inner ear hair cells, was somehow causing tinnitus. However, people have had their hearing nerve surgically cut to try to get rid of tinnitus. The surgery makes a person completely deaf in the ear with the cut nerve since no information coming from the peripheral hearing system can travel up the hearing nerve anymore. After the surgery, people still had tinnitus. More recent brain imaging tests (e.g. Positron-emission tomography or PET Scan) have confirmed tinnitus seems to come from activity in the brain's higher level hearing system.

Because tinnitus likely starts in the brain's hearing system, it is often perceived as coming from both ears or from inside the head. But sometimes people just have tinnitus in one ear. Remember people with tinnitus in one ear only should always get a referral from their family doctor to see an ear specialist, as this type of tinnitus may need medical treatment. Over time, one ear tinnitus often changes to sound as if it is coming from both ears or in the head. The typical reaction for people with this tinnitus is to worry that it has become worse. They fear whatever is wrong with one ear has spread to the other side. What has actually happened is the tinnitus sound message has activated nerve fiber centers high in the hearing system. The tinnitus starts to sound as if it is coming from both ears. When I see clients with tinnitus in one ear, I tell them their tinnitus sound may change to both ears or "in the head" so they shouldn't worry if this happens. I explain that this is a natural way our brains often process tinnitus.

Some researchers make an interesting comparison between tinnitus and phantom limb pain. Tinnitus is the sensation of sound without sound input from the environment. Phantom limb pain is the sensation of pain without physical input. The pain is felt in limbs that are missing (e.g. toes, fingers, legs, arms that are amputated or lost in an accident). Both tinnitus and phantom limb pain happen when there is no input coming from the ear or the limb. Both are generated in the brain. Both are likely related to nerve fiber over-activity that is not suppressed or filtered out by the brain.

Many people distressed by tinnitus are told, "Just don't listen to it". This advice is well meaning but difficult to do in reality. Tinnitus can become recognized as a meaningful sound in the brain the same as the bark of a dog is recognized as a meaningful sound. Try telling yourself that you will never listen to the bark of a dog again. Tell yourself the next time a dog barks that you just won't hear it. I bet you it doesn't work. Obviously you can't just tell yourself not to hear your tinnitus once your brain has already begun processing it as a sound pattern. The good news is that with treatment, it is possible to re-adjust how the brain responds to the patterns of activity heard as tinnitus.

Table 2
HOW TINNITUS IS HEARD

1.	No sound from environment moves through ear system.	**No Sound In**
2.	Nerve fiber over activity starts and sound message is carried through brain.	**Sound Processing**
3.	Tinnitus sound is heard.	

TINNITUS GRIEVANCE

Grievance can be defined as a cause of distress. Tinnitus is certainly distressing for some people. Prolonged tinnitus is present in about 10 to 15% of adults in the general population although it is even more common in adults over age 55. For armed forces personnel with wartime military experience, the percentage having tinnitus rises to around 50%. However, approximately 85% of people who are consciously aware of tinnitus don't find it disturbing or distressing. These people can notice tinnitus when they focus their attention on it, but they are not bothered by it. The remaining people do find their tinnitus bothersome from a mild to severe degree, with a small percentage finding it severely distressing.

J. L. Mayes

Why is tinnitus distressing for some people and not for others? Sound is of great importance to humans. The brain is constantly monitoring our sound environment even when we are unaware of it. The difference between conscious awareness of tinnitus without any distress and awareness of tinnitus with distress depends on a person's reaction to sound. This reaction is largely tied to sound meaning. All sounds have meaning. Some sounds are identified as warning signals. If we hear the sound of a car horn, we may automatically step back on the sidewalk. Other sounds are identified as pleasant like the sound of a loved ones voice or a favourite song. Certain sounds are considered unpleasant like screeching nails on a blackboard. There are many sounds identified as neutral with no negative or positive meaning. These sounds are not liked or disliked; they are just present in our background consciousness. This might include the sound of a fan or refrigerator running.

Sound meaning is different for different people. What may be pleasant for one person may be unpleasant for somebody else. While some people's favourite song might be a great country music tune, other people might hate the very same song. I love the sound of wind chimes. A good friend and colleague of mine hates the sound of wind chimes. She complains regularly about the sound of wind chimes from her neighbour's yard. She has no control over the sound that intrudes on her space. It triggers an unhappy reaction from her.

When sounds have a negative meaning (identified as unpleasant or as a warning), then it is believed these sounds trigger a reaction in what is called the autonomous nervous system of the brain. The autonomous nervous system is responsible for emotion. If a sound (environmental or tinnitus) has no negative emotional meaning, then it can be tuned out or easily ignored. People may be aware but not distressed by it. When my husband and I bought our first home we were thrilled to move in. The first night at 2:00 a.m. we woke up to the sound of train whistles. We hadn't realized that we had moved close to a railway line with a whistle crossing. The trains ran nightly. My husband and I both enjoy the sound of train whistles. To us this sound was not important and was not negative or unpleasant. Although the whistles woke us up the first few nights, within a few weeks, we were sleeping through the night. Our hearing systems were likely still processing the sound as we slept. But it was filtered out so that it never reached our conscious awareness.

If a negative sound travels up the hearing system in the brain, the hearing system may automatically send messages to the emotion system in the brain triggering an emotional reaction. Emotions triggered for negative sounds can include sadness, anger, fear, worry, anxiety or depression. A negative emotional reaction to the sound of train whistles would have activated the hearing system to fully process this sound whenever it happened. This sound would be sent right up the hearing system to consciousness awareness. Sleepless nights and distress would be the result.

A negative emotional reaction increases a sound's importance. Instead of being a meaningless extra "sound message" flowing through the hearing system, tinnitus can become an important sound message both in terms of the hearing system and the emotion system. This reinforces the over-active nerve fiber activity that started the tinnitus sound in the first place. Chronic distressing tinnitus can become established. While the hearing system plays the main role in tinnitus awareness, the emotion system is responsible for whether a person only experiences tinnitus or is distressed by it.

It is not surprising that when tinnitus appears as a new sound signal, it can be identified with a negative sound meaning. It can be as annoying as any other endless or repetitive noise in our environment. If it comes on suddenly, it is more likely to be thought of as a negative sound. Even if it comes on gradually, people often wait years before seeking help. By that time, many people think they are going deaf, going crazy or have a serious medical problem. Unfortunately, when people do seek help for tinnitus, they are usually told there is no cure. Tinnitus is something they just have to learn to live with.

It is difficult to be diagnosed with a chronic condition that is expected to be permanent or long lasting. Many conditions today are fixed with a pill or surgery. When people learn they have something that is not expected to go away and can't be fixed, the initial reaction is often shock and disbelief. People think the diagnosis can't be true. They don't want to believe it. This frequently leads to a search for different medical opinions or treatment answers. There must be somebody or something that can cure this problem. Over a period of weeks, months, or years, people may see various doctors, ear specialists and/or health practitioners trying to find answers.

People soon discover tinnitus can't just be turned off. Once a person realizes that there is no quick fix available, then grief or distress often set in. Grief is associated with feelings of sadness, anger, fear, worry, anxiety and depression. These are the same feelings tinnitus can trigger in the brain's emotion system. So a person's distressing emotional reaction to tinnitus can be both caused by and reinforced by grief. These feelings are a completely normal reaction. But they can also reinforce and aggravate the tinnitus if the negative cycle is kept up. The nerve fibers keep up their work responding to this sound signal. The over active hearing system continues to feed the negative emotional reaction for tinnitus. Tinnitus distress will not improve if this cycle continues:

1. Negative emotional reaction towards tinnitus (e.g. worry, fear, anxiety, sadness, depression).

2. Tinnitus is distressing.

3. Nerve fibers stay over active (tinnitus sound maintained or increased).

4. Repeat from step 1 or use treatment tools to stop the cycle.

There is no difference in tinnitus characteristics between people who just experience tinnitus and those who are distressed by it. One might assume that the most distressed people have the loudest tinnitus. But this is not the case. A person can have loud tinnitus with no distress. Another person can have soft tinnitus with great distress. In fact it is possible to find two people with identical loudness and pitch of tinnitus and identical hearing, but one person will be able to ignore the tinnitus and the other person will be very bothered by it.

It is not the tinnitus sound itself that causes distress. It is the person's reaction to the tinnitus that causes distress. A person can ignore sounds and carry on with their day. Or, a person can easily fall into the negative tinnitus cycle. This negative reaction can be mild to moderate such as occasional frustration or annoyance in specific situations (e.g. noticing tinnitus when trying to read or fall asleep). The reaction can also be severe enough to overwhelm a person's daily life. Difficulties with sleep, concentration, and relaxation are common. In very severe cases, tinnitus distress can affect a person's whole life including home, work and social situations.

For most people, emotions are reflected in their thoughts. We all have a running stream of thoughts in our heads. This background flow is typically made up of random thoughts that pop in our heads as we go through our day. Thoughts can cover anything and everything from shopping lists, to-do lists, secret opinions, worries and dreams. Background thoughts can be called our inner voice. This voice is always there. This voice is a good reflection of how a person is reacting to their tinnitus. When a person has a negative reaction to their tinnitus, then typical thoughts might include:

•   What if I have a serious illness?

- What if the tinnitus gets worse?

- What if I lose my hearing?

- What if I can never enjoy peace and quiet?

- What if I can't work?

- What if I can't live with it?

As Mark Twain once said, "I am an old man and have had many troubles, most of which never happened". "What if" thinking can create unfounded tinnitus troubles. If a person with tinnitus is given correct information when they seek help, these thoughts can often be nipped in the bud. If these thoughts are allowed to fester, then increased tinnitus distress is far more likely.

SOUND SENSITIVITY

For some people, a negative emotional reaction can also affect the hearing system for regular everyday sounds. Normal sounds in our environment start to be experienced as uncomfortably loud. Typical daily sounds like doors closing, running water, cooking noises or normal conversation cause pain or discomfort. It is as if the volume of the world is stuck on high. The most common technical term for sound sensitivity is "hyperacusis", although other terms may also be used (e.g. phonophobia, misophonia, etc.). People may start to fear and dislike sound when it becomes uncomfortable to hear. This fear and dislike can be for specific sounds or for sounds in general. Sound sensitivity often develops after an event that triggers a strong emotional reaction.

Case 11: He developed sound sensitivity after a co-worker surprised him by setting off a firecracker right behind him as a joke.

Case 12: She developed sound sensitivity after a severe head injury.

Researchers believe sound sensitivity comes from the brain's hearing system pathways. It is thought the hearing system turns up the intensity or loudness for sounds that were once entirely comfortable. Remember how the hearing system processes sound and silence. It seems nerve fiber networks can become over-active for sound as well as for silence. With tinnitus, nerve fiber activity is amplified and processed as sound. With sound sensitivity, nerve fiber activity is amplified and processed as increased sound.

Table 3
HOW SOUND SENSITIVITY HAPPENS

1. Sound from environment moves through ear system.	**Sound In**
2. Nerve fiber over activity starts and increased sound message is carried through brain.	**Sound Processing**
3. Increased sound is heard.	

Sounds processed in the auditory pathways are heard louder than they actually are. Almost half of people with sound sensitivity also have tinnitus. Both tinnitus and sound sensitivity appear to have similar origins in the brain's hearing system. As with tinnitus, sound sensitivity will not improve if a cycle of reacting negatively towards sound continues:

1. Negative emotional reaction towards sound (e.g. worry, fear, anxiety, sadness, depression).

2. Sound sensitivity is distressing.

3. Nerve fibers stay over active (sound sensitivity maintained or increased).

4. Repeat from step 1 or use treatment tools to stop the cycle.

CHANGING REACTIONS

Unfortunately, people with tinnitus (or sound sensitivity) often react by avoiding sound. They may try to stay in quiet environments or even start using earplugs or earmuffs to protect themselves from potentially loud sounds they might encounter in their daily life. This lowers input flowing through the hearing system. This increases nerve fiber activity. Increased nerve fiber activity can then cause increased tinnitus or sound sensitivity. Sound avoidance will not help the negative emotional reaction of tinnitus distress and/or sound sensitivity. As a result, tinnitus or sound sensitivity can easily worsen if not treated appropriately. If people with tinnitus also have sound sensitivity, both must be treated to get best results.

In terms of treatment, it is important to understand that a person's emotional reaction to tinnitus or sound can be changed. The following is an example of how an emotional reaction to an event can be completely switched over time. I live in Vancouver, British Columbia, Canada. This area has a large number of illegal marijuana growing operations. These drug homes are typically based in residential neighbourhoods. Rival criminals often target them for drive by shootings and armed robbery invasions. The most common sign of a marijuana grow operation is a house where windows stay covered day and night, and no activity is seen from the outside. We once lived next to a house where we never saw our neighbour. Window coverings were always closed. Only very occasionally would someone enter or exit the home, and this was usually very early in the morning or late at night.

We began to worry. Had we moved next to a drug house? What if there was a drive-by shooting? What if our family or our house was targeted by mistake? We became very aware of any activity next door. We watched anxiously, extremely worried about a potentially dangerous situation. This worry began to intrude on our lives, and became an ongoing topic of discussion. One day we were talking with a different neighbour. We found out that the owner of the house next door was extremely shy and did not like being outdoors. She worked long hours. When she was at home, she enjoyed staying indoors and spending time with her cat. There was zero possibility that she was growing drugs. Our anxiety and fear disappeared. Nothing had changed about our next-door neighbour or her home situation. But our reaction was no longer negative.

With appropriate treatment, negative emotional reactions can be changed for any degree of tinnitus distress. Information on how treatment is modified to help sound sensitivity is also discussed in this book. Changing how you react to tinnitus (or sound) can be as difficult as learning to write with your left hand if you are right handed. The good news is that using appropriate techniques, the emotional meaning of tinnitus or sound can be altered so that it becomes of little or no importance. The sound itself may remain completely unchanged. But the distress connection between the hearing system and the emotion system in the brain can be reset. Dramatic improvement in coping can happen when a person changes their reaction. Specific techniques are available that have been used successfully by many people. Keep in mind that the longer the distress or sensitivity has been present, the longer it will take to see positive changes. Changing your reaction can't happen overnight. But it can happen.

TINNITUS EVALUATION

Nothing happens to any man that he is not formed by nature to bear. Marcus Aurelius.

Because tinnitus is associated with so many conditions, it is important to have a family doctor and/or ear specialist (e.g. Otologist or Otolaryngologist) evaluation to see if medical treatment is needed. The medical evaluation typically happens before the tinnitus evaluation. Further medical follow-up may also be recommended after the tinnitus evaluation depending on findings. These are standard routine referrals. Sometimes medical examination and testing (e.g. CT Scan, Magnetic Resonance Imaging or MRI, etc.) is required. In the vast majority of cases, these tests don't demonstrate any specific problem.

Many people hope to pinpoint what caused their tinnitus believing this will lead to a cure for them. But in the majority of cases, their doctor or ear specialist will not find any specific cause. After medical evaluation, people are often told there is nothing that can be done for their tinnitus. It is true that often there is no need for medical treatment. Even in cases where medical treatment is needed for a health condition associated with tinnitus, that treatment will not necessarily make the tinnitus disappear. But anyone with tinnitus can certainly benefit from tinnitus treatment. The focus of tinnitus treatment is to decrease any distress and improve quality of life.

The tinnitus evaluation is the first step towards an individual tinnitus treatment plan. Audiologists or tinnitus specialists usually do tinnitus evaluations. Audiologists are professionals with specialized training in non-medical treatment for ear problems including tinnitus. Tinnitus specialists are professionals (often audiologists) with specialized training in specific types of tinnitus or sound sensitivity treatment. Audiologists have training and experience in hearing problems, how the hearing system works, hearing testing, hearing related devices, and counselling. They are also able to make referrals to ear specialists, tinnitus specialists or other professionals when needed. Most people with distressing tinnitus will benefit from a team approach involving at least their family doctor, ear specialist, and audiologist or tinnitus specialist. Other counselling specialists (e.g. psychologist, psychiatrist or other mental health professional) can also be of great help for people with severe tinnitus distress.

The challenge with tinnitus evaluation is that there are currently no set evaluation guidelines. Tinnitus evaluation can vary from clinic to clinic and from care provider to care provider. Researchers are working towards developing a standard clinical evaluation procedure for people with tinnitus. Currently, many experts recommend that a tinnitus evaluation with an audiologist should include an interview, hearing assessment, tinnitus assessment, sound sensitivity assessment (if necessary), tinnitus questionnaires, and education and reassurance counselling.

This chapter explains each of these components of a tinnitus evaluation. Evaluation components actually used will vary on a case-by-case basis depending on the individual person and the clinic they go to. A person seeing a tinnitus specialist at a tinnitus clinic will likely receive all these components. A person seeing an audiologist at a hearing clinic may not. The goal of this chapter is for people to better understand how tinnitus and sound sensitivity may be evaluated. The biggest factor in determining whether tinnitus or sound sensitivity is a problem requiring treatment is the information you give the care provider on how it is affecting your daily life.

Information is presented in an order for ease of understanding, and is not the order of information gathering and testing necessarily used in a clinical setting. Also specific tinnitus evaluation components may change over time as more is learned about tinnitus and as new treatment approaches become available.

Keep in mind that tinnitus evaluation involves directing your attention on your tinnitus. This typically starts before the appointment as people rehearse what they want to share with their care provider. Throughout the appointment people are focusing on their tinnitus and straining to hear during testing. During the interview and counselling there is much discussion about the person's hearing, tinnitus and any related concerns. The common result is a temporary worsening of tinnitus after the tinnitus evaluation appointment. What you focus on increases. This is a completely normal and natural occurrence that can also occur after hearing testing alone. Over time (often within a day or two) the tinnitus will settle back to its usual state.

INTERVIEW

Interview questions will vary from clinic to clinic depending on the evaluation approach being used. Care providers will typically ask questions about your medical history, your tinnitus, and any effect tinnitus is having on your quality of life.

There are various conditions that are associated with the symptom of tinnitus. The development of these conditions can also trigger increased tinnitus in someone who already has tinnitus. People with tinnitus should expect to be asked for detailed information about their medical history when they are seen for a tinnitus evaluation. This information can help the care provider identify potential tinnitus causes or triggers. However, in most cases no specific cause comes to light. You may be asked about your general health and any medical conditions that you have; any prescription medications or supplements that you are taking; imbalance or dizziness; ear pain, infection or surgery; family history of hearing loss; noise exposure (military, work or hobbies); gunfire or firearm exposure; as well as any history of head injury with concussion or loss of consciousness.

People are usually asked for a detailed description of their tinnitus to help plan testing, counselling and treatment. You may be asked if you feel distress or not; what the tinnitus sounds like; where you hear it (e.g. in left ear, in head); how and when it started; how often you hear it; what the loudness is like (e.g. stable, variable); if the loudness ever changes because of sounds around you; and if regular everyday sounds are ever bothersome or unpleasant.

There is a proper way to finding out if a person is distressed by their tinnitus. The care provider should ask very general questions rather than negatively phrased questions such as "How much does your tinnitus bother you?" which leads a person into thinking their tinnitus should bother them. Remember a large percentage of people are not at all distressed by their tinnitus. A common question used by many care providers is "How do you feel about your tinnitus?" When I ask this question in my clinic I get two types of answers. Either people say they are used to it, or there is often a long pause and then people start talking about the difficulties they are having. So there may be no concerns, concerns in specific situations, or widespread concerns in daily activities.

If you are distressed, then the focus is finding out what it is about the tinnitus that makes it distressing. Part of this is finding out how you react to changes in tinnitus loudness. It is completely normal and natural for tinnitus to fluctuate on its own in loudness over time. Some people start tinnitus diaries to track their diet, sleep cycles, etc. to try to find a link between their daily lifestyle and their tinnitus loudness. These types of tinnitus diaries are typically counterproductive because they focus attention on tinnitus, which can increase distress. People also often end up very frustrated when they can't pinpoint any consistent cause for tinnitus loudness variation. This is because tinnitus naturally changes in loudness on its own without cause. How you react to natural tinnitus loudness changes influences the amount of distress experienced. The treatment needed depends on the distress present.

It is also helpful to find out if sounds around you ever make your tinnitus loudness change or if you find the loudness of everyday sounds bothersome. It is normal to notice changes in tinnitus loudness after exposure to very loud sounds. Treatment must take into consideration any exposure to noise loud enough to damage the ears. Some people report concerns about the loudness of regular everyday sounds. This can indicate potential sound sensitivity that also needs to be addressed in treatment.

HEARING ASSESSMENT

Many people with tinnitus have some hearing loss present. Many people also think it is their tinnitus that makes it hard for them to hear. Hearing and communication problems are not caused by tinnitus. They are caused by hearing loss. Because hearing loss is so common in people with tinnitus, anyone with tinnitus should have their hearing tested. A thorough hearing assessment is a key component of a tinnitus evaluation. Treatment must address tinnitus as well as any hearing loss present. On-line hearing tests are not accurate and should never be used. People with tinnitus should only have their hearing evaluated by a qualified care provider (e.g. audiologist).

Hearing testing should be done inside a sound proof booth to get accurate results. Each ear is tested individually, although some testing may be done with signals sent to both ears. Most hearing testing is done using an audiometer. An audiometer is a machine used to test hearing status. The audiometer sends signals to the ear. Different signals can be used including tones, speech, or noise.

Frequency (pitch) and intensity (loudness) of different signals are adjusted as needed during testing. Hearing assessment done as part of a tinnitus evaluation usually includes a visual check of the ears, pure tone testing, speech testing, middle ear testing, and inner ear testing.

Visual check of the ears is done before testing. Care providers should routinely look inside their client's ears using an otoscope. This is a device that provides specialized lighting for a visual check of the ear canals and eardrum. This visual check can pick up problems (e.g. unexpected objects sitting in the ear canal, inflammation, infection, scarring or holes in the eardrum, etc.). It can also detect any excess earwax in the ear canal or sitting on the eardrum (which can cause tinnitus). If there is too much earwax present, then it should be safely removed by a qualified professional (e.g. ear specialist, family doctor or audiologist trained and experienced in this procedure). Cleaning by irrigation or by sending water down the ear canal wall can be too loud for some people with tinnitus or sound sensitivity. If necessary, ideally your care provider is willing to use other available less noisy methods to help reduce or remove earwax. The size and shape of the ear canal is also inspected since this may affect fit of any recommended devices.

Pure tone testing checks the peripheral hearing system (outer, middle and inner ears). With pure tone testing, tones are presented at different intensities (loudness) measured in decibels (dB) across a standard frequency (pitch) range. Typically the frequency range tested is 250 to 8000 Hz since this is the most important range for speech communication. Threshold is defined as the softest intensity a person can hear a pure tone at a specific frequency. People with thresholds of 20 to 25 dB or less across 250 to 8000 Hz have normal hearing.

Pure tone thresholds are typically obtained using air conduction and bone conduction signals. Air conduction signals are usually presented through insert phones (foam "plugs" that go in the ears). Sometimes earphones ("muffs" on the ears) may be used. Sound signals travel through air (down the ear canal and through the middle ear system) to get to the inner ear. Bone conduction signals are presented through a special vibrator usually placed behind the ear or on the forehead. Sound signals bypass the middle ear system by traveling through bone (of the skull) to get to the inner ear.

Pure tone testing will identify whether there is hearing loss at any frequency. If hearing loss is present, a comparison of air and bone conduction thresholds will identify whether the hearing loss is from a problem with the outer and/

or middle ear (conductive hearing loss), a problem with the inner ear (sensorineural hearing loss) or a combination of conductive and sensorineural components (mixed hearing loss). If any conductive hearing loss is present, then a referral to an ear specialist is needed to see if medical treatment is possible (if you haven't seen an ear specialist already).

For pure tone testing, people are typically told they will hear a series of soft beeps or notes. They are asked to respond (lift a finger or press a button) when they hear a sound even when it is very faint or far away. This is where people with tinnitus may get frustrated. Many people with tinnitus are considered "difficult to test" when having their hearing tested, because they have difficulty distinguishing between their tinnitus and the test signals being presented. They respond to test signals and they respond to "nothing" when they mistake their tinnitus for the test tones.

Typical test tones are a series of beeps lasting approximately 3 seconds for each beep presented (e.g. beeeeeep). This type of beep often sounds similar to a person's tinnitus especially at certain pitches or frequencies. However, audiometer settings can be changed from continuous to pulsed tones. Pulsed tones are a series of short pulsed tones (e.g. bip bip bip) presented for approximately 3 seconds for each series presented. Research has demonstrated that thresholds are the same for pulsed and continuous tones. Using pulsed tones can help some patients better tell when they are hearing a test tone and not their tinnitus. It is recommended that people with tinnitus request pulsed tones for pure tone threshold testing if their care provider is not already using this presentation method.

Author's Case: I hate having my hearing tested. I hear lots of beeps and rings inside my head. When I sit in a soundproof booth (very quiet environment) and listen hard for test tones, my tinnitus takes off. I have often had the care provider walk into the booth (while obviously no test signal is being sent) as I sat pressing away in response to my own tinnitus. When I have my hearing tested, I request the use of pulsed tones to help me better distinguish test tones from my tinnitus.

In the past, I constantly noticed the same problem with clients. I began using pulsed tones when testing clients with tinnitus. I check if my client's tinnitus sounds like the pulsed type tone I will be using. In the vast majority of cases the pulsed tone is sufficiently different from their tinnitus. I can then instruct my clients to try to respond only to pulsed tones, but not for other type sounds. I find my clients with tinnitus perform much better in detecting true test signals from their tinnitus when I use this pulsed tone technique. As a result, I now routinely use pulsed tones during testing for all my clients.

If hearing loss is found with pure tone testing, the loss is typically described by type (conductive, sensorineural or mixed) and by severity. It is not appropriate to use percentages to describe the amount of hearing loss present. Severity descriptions are used instead (e.g. mild, moderate, moderately severe, severe or profound). Severity often varies across the frequency range. For example, a person may have normal low frequency hearing sloping to a moderately severe high frequency hearing loss in both ears. The type, severity and frequency pattern of hearing loss present is unrelated to tinnitus distress. People with distressing tinnitus may have any type or pattern of hearing loss ranging from mild to profound.

Speech testing usually includes two parts: speech thresholds and word recognition testing. For speech thresholds, standardized lists of easy two syllable words (e.g. airplane, baseball, sunshine) are presented at different intensities or loudness levels. Threshold is defined as the softest intensity (loudness) a person can hear and repeat back the words. Many people end up memorizing these words after having their hearing tested more than once. You are supposed to be familiar with the words used. Some care providers will even go through the list with you before starting. Since there are multiple words and they would not be presented in the same order each time, this is not a problem. Thresholds from test to test would still be accurate. Speech is made up of a combination of pure tones, so speech thresholds should be consistent with pure tone thresholds. Speech threshold testing helps double check reliability of pure tone responses.

For word recognition testing, standardized lists of one syllable words (e.g. chew, knees) are presented at the person's most comfortable listening level. The lists are designed to pick up common mistakes in distinguishing words made by people with hearing loss. For example, a person might hear "knees" as "knee" or "me". Although people with tinnitus often have their hearing tested on multiple occasions, there is not any concern that a person might memorize these lists as a way of improving their results. Providers select from multiple standardized lists with varying words and word order used from test to test. Presentation is usually at a person's preferred most comfortable loudness level. Usually 25 to 50 words are presented to each ear although a shorter 10-word list may be used in a hearing screening. Results are reported as the percentage of words repeated correctly. Word recognition can be described as excellent, good, fair, poor, or extremely poor.

People with conductive hearing loss typically have good word recognition once words are presented at sufficient loudness. People with sensorineural hearing loss often still have good word recognition at louder listening levels. Significantly impaired word recognition indicates the presence of built-in distortion within the hearing system. A large unexplained difference in word recognition between ears usually requires medical referral to an ear specialist. If treating hearing loss, hearing aids can't correct for built-in distortion although they can still be helpful in balancing hearing between the ears. Counselling on realistic expectations is an important aspect of hearing aid fitting for people with impaired word recognition results.

Case 13: He reported tinnitus that he thought interfered with his hearing. He could hear when people were talking but sometimes couldn't make out the words. Results showed severe high frequency sensorineural hearing loss with good to excellent word recognition scores of 84% in the left ear and 96% in the right ear (presented at a louder than conversational listening levels). He would be a good hearing aid candidate in both ears.

Case 14: She reported tinnitus and great difficulty hearing in her right ear after a stroke. Group situations were particularly difficult. She had seen an ear specialist, and no further medical evaluation or treatment was planned. She was referred for evaluation with an audiologist. Results showed a mild high frequency sensorineural hearing loss in the left ear with excellent word recognition (100%), and a severe sensorineural hearing loss across the frequency range in the right ear with extremely poor word recognition (20%). She would be a good hearing aid candidate in the left ear, but right ear hearing aid benefit would be limited because of the built-in distortion.

Case 15: She had repeated ear infections throughout her life along with tinnitus in both ears. Results showed moderate bilateral conductive hearing loss with excellent word recognition (100% in the right ear and 96% in the left ear). She was referred to an ear specialist to see if medical treatment was possible before considering hearing aids.

Middle ear testing is used to identify any problems with the middle ear system. The middle ear system is made up of the eardrum and middle ear bones. Testing is done using a machine that can do tympanometry (testing of eardrum movement and pressure status) and acoustic reflexes (testing of middle ear bone movement). For these tests, a plug is placed in the person's ear and they are asked to sit very still without moving. The machine does all the testing automatically without any response from the person being tested. Testing does not need to be done in a sound proof booth.

For eardrum testing, the person feels a sensation of pressure. This test shows how the eardrum is moving and how it is sitting within the ear canal. It can detect holes or other problems with the eardrum. A stiff eardrum movement can be from a problem like a middle ear infection (e.g. fluid sitting behind the eardrum stops it from moving properly). An overly mobile eardrum movement can be from a healed hole in the eardrum or from a dislocation of the middle ear bones behind the eardrum. This test is very useful in combination with other hearing tests used in a hearing evaluation.

For acoustic reflex testing, extremely loud beeps are used to trigger a very small muscle reflex that pulls on the stirrup (stapes) middle ear bone. When the middle ear system is "hit" by loud sound, the muscle to the bone contracts reflexively. This reflex is similar to the patellar reflex that doctors check when they hit below the kneecap to see if they can make your leg kick out. The acoustic reflex is either present or absent. When it is present, it indicates that the middle ear bones are moving adequately in response to loud sound. When it is absent, this result is often inconclusive. It can mean the plug placed in the ear is not sealing off the ear canal well enough to pick up this small reflex. It can indicate a problem within the middle ear system. It can indicate a hearing loss of any type is present.

Acoustic reflex testing is not recommended for people with tinnitus for several reasons. Results are often inconclusive. Middle ear system status can be evaluated using other tests (e.g. eardrum testing, comparison of air and bone conduction hearing thresholds, etc.). Also, many people with tinnitus have some sound sensitivity. They are often made uncomfortable by the extreme loudness of tones used to trigger the acoustic reflex.

Author's Case: As a person with tinnitus as well as an audiologist, I consider acoustic reflex testing unnecessary for people with tinnitus. Before I do middle ear testing, I explain to my clients that I am going to check their eardrum and it may feel strange. I also explain that some clinics do an extra acoustic reflex test with very loud sounds. I let my clients know that I never use that loud test on anyone with tinnitus. I explain I can get the same information through a combination of other hearing tests. I encourage them to request "no acoustic reflex testing" if they are seen at a different clinic.

Case 16: He was seen for hearing loss and tinnitus. The audiologist explained that acoustic reflex testing would not be done so he would not be subjected to loud sounds. He told them "Just go ahead. Do what you have to do. I can take it." The audiologist explained that there was no valid reason to do this test, and they could get all the information they needed without it. He appreciated that testing was customized for his tinnitus needs.

Case 17: She was seen for tinnitus and sound sensitivity. She was nervous about the type of sounds that would be used for testing. The audiologist explained that acoustic reflex testing would not be done so she would not be subjected to loud sounds. She became more relaxed. She was grateful that the goal was to use test procedures below her loudness discomfort zone.

Inner ear testing is not available at all hearing clinics. An inner ear or otoacoustic emissions test is used to check peripheral hearing system status. In very simple terms, testing is done using a machine that sends signals down the ear canal, through the middle ear system and to the inner ear. The machine then measures any response or emission from the inner ear. A plug is placed in the person's ear and the person is asked to sit very still without moving. Soft tones are presented across a range of frequencies from low pitch to high pitch. Testing needs to be done in a quiet environment so ambient room noise doesn't cover up responses.

If a response is present at a given frequency, it typically indicates a normal middle ear system and good hearing (at worst no more than a mild hearing loss present). Absent responses may indicate the presence of hearing loss. The pattern of emissions across the frequency range typically matches the pattern of any hearing loss across the frequency range for pure tone testing. Responses can also be hidden if there is too much background noise present in the room. While absent otoacoustic emissions can be inconclusive, the presence of these emissions can provide helpful information about inner ear status.

Otoacoustic emissions testing can be a helpful replacement for acoustic reflex testing. Although these emissions don't test the middle ear bones directly, any problem with the middle ear system can result in absent emissions. This can support information about conductive hearing loss obtained from eardrum testing and a comparison of air and bone conduction hearing thresholds.

> **Case 18:** She had tinnitus and normal hearing. Otoacoustic emissions were present and robust at all frequencies. This information was used during counselling to reassure her about the health of her outer, middle and inner ears. She was more open to learning about the central mechanism for tinnitus within the brain.

> **Case 19:** This man had tinnitus and moderate high frequency sensorineural hearing loss. Otoacoustic emissions were present in the low frequencies, but absent in the high frequencies. In combination, all hearing evaluation results demonstrated the presence of inner ear related hearing loss and no middle ear problems. Treatment for tinnitus and hearing loss was recommended.

TINNITUS ASSESSMENT

There is currently no clinical test that can directly measure tinnitus. While there are many aspects of the human body that can be measured with a test (e.g. cholesterol levels, lung function, hearing, vision), there are other processes that can't be directly measured (e.g. pain levels). A person may tell their doctor that they have a terrible headache or severe back pain. But there is no way to directly measure this. In the same way, there is currently no test that can measure the severity of a person's tinnitus. Just like pain, tinnitus severity can only be judged indirectly. People report what their tinnitus sounds like and whether their quality of life is affected by it. Further detail on tinnitus characteristics can be obtained through the tinnitus assessment. This helps identify treatment needs, although it may not be done unless you go to a tinnitus specialist. Usually tinnitus assessment includes matching measurements and measurement of the effect sound has on the tinnitus. Tinnitus questionnaires are also often used.

Tinnitus matching measurements help check the reported pitch and loudness of a person's tinnitus. Some people find it very reassuring that their internal sound which nobody else can hear can be compared to a real world sound. Matching is usually done in the ear with the loudest tinnitus. If tinnitus is fairly equal between ears, then it doesn't matter which ear is used. For tinnitus matching, a person is asked to compare their tinnitus to a tone or noise presented through the audiometer. The pitch (frequency) and loudness (intensity) is adjusted as necessary until the best approximate match to the person's tinnitus is found. Typically a pitch match is obtained first, and then a loudness match is obtained at the tinnitus pitch match.

For pitch matches, most people with tinnitus will select a matching pitch in the high frequency range. When hearing loss is present, the tinnitus pitch matches may be at or close to the frequency of greatest hearing loss although this is not always the case. It is common for pitch matches to vary from appointment to appointment.

Loudness matches are measured at the tinnitus pitch match. They tend to be fairly consistent over time. People with normal hearing typically select somewhat louder matches than people with hearing loss. Loudness matches in general are slightly above hearing thresholds. Often the loudness match is within 10 dB of a person's hearing threshold at a particular pitch match. For example, a person's hearing threshold might be at 60 dB, and their tinnitus loudness match at 65 dB. Some people are surprised to learn that their tinnitus loudness match is close to their hearing threshold, which does not seem to match up to their perception of an extremely loud tinnitus sound. This may be incorrectly interpreted to suggest that their tinnitus sound is soft or faint. Measurements in dB can somewhat underestimate perceived loudness. This is because dB is an intensity scale. The scale used for subjective loudness is the sone scale. Most care providers will not do the calculation to convert dB into sone. The main point to keep in mind is that a person's tinnitus can certainly sound loud regardless of the loudness match.

In some tinnitus clinics, the effect of sound on tinnitus is measured since sound is an important component of treatment. The Minimum Masking Level (MML) is the softest level of noise needed so a person can no longer hear their tinnitus. The type of noise used is broadband or white noise where the noise is made up of all frequencies, with equal sound energy at each frequency. It sounds like a "shhhhh" type sound. The noise is usually presented to both ears if tinnitus is in both ears and to one ear if the tinnitus is in one ear. MMLs help indicate how helpful sound will be in making a person's tinnitus less noticeable, and how much sound might be required. Some people have tinnitus that is more easily covered up than others. Some people may need more sound than others in treatment. MML results help guide what treatment approach may be most effective for each individual.

Some care providers may do an additional residual inhibition test to measure if a person's tinnitus changes after white noise is presented for a certain period of time and then turned off. The tinnitus may become softer or disappear during this test. The effect is usually very short, lasting only up to a few seconds to a few minutes in most people. Mainly this test shows whether a person's tinnitus is responsive to noise. It can be used to help demonstrate to people that sound can be beneficial in treating their tinnitus.

Tinnitus questionnaires are commonly used as part of a comprehensive tinnitus evaluation. Various questionnaires are available that have been assessed by the scientific community for reliability and consistency. However, there is currently no single tinnitus questionnaire in universal clinical use. Questionnaires contain standardized lists of questions. The questions are designed to identify problem areas that may be present if a person is distressed by their tinnitus. Questions may target emotions (e.g. anger, frustration, depression, anxiety), limitations (e.g. difficulty with concentration, reading, sleep, household responsibilities, work, social activities) and inability to cope (e.g. desperation, loss of control, inability to escape).

Questionnaires are scored. Based on the questionnaire score, people are typically divided into tinnitus severity categories that may range from no problem to mild, moderate, or severe tinnitus distress. Typically, the more distressed a person is by their tinnitus, the more widespread the problem areas identified through the questionnaire, and the greater the perceived severity of the tinnitus. Questionnaires in combination with the tinnitus evaluation interview are very helpful in identifying problems areas and in planning treatment. Questionnaire results can identify pre-treatment perceived tinnitus severity. People can then repeat these written questionnaires during and at the end of treatment. Any changes in results can be used to evaluate treatment effectiveness over time. With successful treatment, people should improve in their ability to cope with tinnitus. Reduced tinnitus severity scores on these standardized questionnaires should reflect this.

Informal severity ranking scales are another method sometimes used for people with tinnitus. People are typically asked to rank their perceived tinnitus severity on a scale of 1 to 10. They may also be asked to rank each particular component of tinnitus distress (e.g. concentration, sleep, anxiety) on a scale of 1 to 10. These types of informal ranking scales are mainly used because they are easy and fast for people to complete. However, when these types of scales are used alone (without any other questionnaires) they are not specific or detailed enough to highlight key concerns or to allow for comparison of treatment progress over time. An additional concern is that a scale of 1 to 10 is often not wide enough to account for day-to-day fluctuations. If a person rates their tinnitus as 10 (most distressing) and everyday it is at a 10, this does little to ease distress or remove attention from the tinnitus. If a scale of 1 to 100 is used, this often gives a wide enough scale to reflect even small changes in tinnitus distress over time. If informal ranking scales are used, a scale of 1 to 100 is recommended.

SOUND SENSITIVITY ASSESSMENT

This testing is completed if sound sensitivity is reported as a concern, although it may only be done if you go to a tinnitus specialist. It is important to distinguish between loudness recruitment and sound sensitivity. People with sensorineural hearing loss often report discomfort to loud sounds. They commonly find that while they can't hear soft sounds properly, they can still hear and be bothered by loud sounds (e.g. a fire alarm) that also sound loud to family and friends. People sometimes assume that when hearing loss is present, all sounds will be muffled. However, people with sensorineural hearing loss often still have normal loudness perception for intense sounds despite having hearing loss for softer sounds. This is called loudness recruitment. It is a normal and natural effect in people with sensorineural hearing loss.

In contrast, sound sensitivity typically refers to discomfort or pain from ordinary everyday sounds not found loud or uncomfortable by other people (e.g. doors closing, water running, normal conversation, etc.). If a person reports concerns that they are bothered by everyday sounds around them, then Loudness Discomfort Level (LDL) testing may be conducted. LDLs are checked across frequencies to find when sounds become uncomfortable. At each frequency or pitch, the person is asked to listen to tones as the intensity or loudness is increased in very small steps. People are typically asked to let the care provider know when the loudness would be ok for a few seconds but not for longer. If LDLs are lower than normal (e.g. loudness would not be ok for regular everyday sound intensities), then a person may have sound sensitivity.

Some people find it reassuring that his or her comfort range can be checked with real world sounds. But the levels obtained are less important than the person's reported discomfort problems in daily life. Counselling and treatment planning must address any sound sensitivity present.

EDUCATION AND REASSURANCE COUNSELLING

Counselling and treatment should try to address any concerns reported during the interview and evaluation. At the end of a tinnitus evaluation, the care provider should have a good understanding of their client's needs and concerns. Is further referral to a doctor or ear specialist needed? Is hearing loss a concern? Is tinnitus a concern? Is sound sensitivity a concern? Is hazardous noise exposure a concern? It is then very important that the care provider spends time on counselling. This counselling should cover education, reassurance, and treatment recommendations. Education is usually given on:

- How we hear.
- How we hear tinnitus.
- How tinnitus is a benign, natural symptom.
- How tinnitus distress relates to how we react to tinnitus rather than the characteristics of the tinnitus itself.
- If present, how sound sensitivity is a benign symptom that relates to how we react to sound.
- What your evaluation results showed.
- What treatment, if any, would be appropriate for your concerns.

The provider should also give reassurance. A person may already be using appropriate coping strategies that they should continue. The provider might also recommend fine-tuning or altering strategies for better benefit. In some cases, a person might be reassured that they don't need any further treatment. In other cases, people can be reassured that there are helpful coping strategies and treatments available.

If there are potential medical issues identified, the person will need to see their doctor or ear specialist. Referrals may be made for other hearing or balance system testing as needed. Two additional tests that are sometimes used are Electronystagmography and Auditory Brainstem Response testing. Electronystagmography (ENG) is a specialized balance system test. It involves sending water into the ears, and it can be loud. Auditory Brainstem Response testing (ABR) is a specialized hearing system test used to check how sound is processed along the hearing or auditory nerve. This test uses very loud sound. Sometimes there are alternative tests that can be used (e.g. CT Scan, Magnetic Resonance Imaging or MRI, etc.). CT Scans and particularly MRIs can also be loud. But people may be able to use hearing protection during these tests (e.g. MRI-safe hearing protection). Speak to your doctor or ear specialist if you are concerned about the loudness of any test. Sometimes other acceptable tests may be available that are quieter or are a test where people can use hearing protection during testing.

If any hearing loss is present, then hearing loss management is essential. If a person is distressed, the treatment is planned based on whether the issue is tinnitus alone or tinnitus with hearing loss and/or sound sensitivity. Tinnitus treatment must also take into consideration whether a person is exposed to hazardous noise during work or hobbies. Appropriate use of hearing protection is an important component of treatment in many cases. Maintaining a healthy lifestyle (e.g. diet, exercise, sleep) is also important for anyone with tinnitus or sound sensitivity.

If tinnitus treatment is recommended, then the provider can review options and make recommendations based on your individual needs. The final decision whether to proceed with treatment rests with you. You must be motivated to follow recommendations, use any recommended devices, and make changes in your daily life. Tinnitus treatment will not give a "quick fix" or cure. But over time an individual treatment plan can certainly lower distress and improve your quality of life.

TREATMENT PLANNING

When one door closes, another opens; but we often look so regretfully upon the closed door that we do not see the one that has been opened for us. Alexander Graham Bell.

Treatment may include medical and/or tinnitus specific treatment. In case there is a medically treatable cause, it is recommended you obtain the approval of your doctor and/or ear specialist before you begin a tinnitus treatment plan. The focus of medical treatment is to correct or manage any medical conditions present. The focus of tinnitus treatment is to decrease any tinnitus distress present and improve quality of life. Tinnitus treatment can happen alone or in combination with medical treatment depending on the individual person.

MEDICAL TREATMENT

Tinnitus has been linked with various ear and medical conditions. Ear conditions can include outer ear problems, middle ear problems or inner ear problems. Outer ear problems can include infections, earwax, etc. Middle ear problems can include infections, dislocated or fractured middle ear bones, Otosclerosis (bony build-up on middle ear bones), etc. Inner ear problems can be due to hearing loss including from age, noise, infection, Meniere's, meningitis, labyrinthitis, toxic drugs, etc.

Medical conditions include head or neck injury (e.g. whiplash, concussion or skull fracture), cardiovascular disease (e.g. heart conditions, stroke, vascular or arterial problems, etc), thyroid disease, diabetes, anemia, dental or jaw problems, etc. Tinnitus can appear after surgery. Tinnitus is also a side effect of many drugs or medications. In some people, it has been suggested tinnitus is related to stress or even genetic predisposition. There is a higher incidence of tinnitus in people with chronic pain or migraines. Tinnitus has also been linked with food allergies and mercury (amalgam) teeth fillings. Because tinnitus is associated with so many things, some people wonder if it is more correct to ask, "What doesn't cause tinnitus?"

Sound sensitivity is linked with various conditions also common to tinnitus. These can include noise exposure, hearing loss, ear conditions, head or neck injury, dental or jaw problems, reaction to medications or surgery, etc. As with tinnitus, the cause of sound sensitivity is often unknown.

If a person has ear, medical, or dental conditions, then they must work with the appropriate health care professionals to treat these conditions. Maximizing health will also maximize coping. If medical treatment includes prescription drugs, then be aware that many prescription drugs can cause or worsen tinnitus in some people. If you are taking prescription drugs to help you cope (e.g. for sleep, anxiety or depression), the same concern applies. Ironically, some of the drugs prescribed for tinnitus (e.g. antidepressants) can make tinnitus worse as a side effect or withdrawal symptom. In addition, it has been found that the effective dose for treating tinnitus is often well below that usually used for treating the general population without tinnitus. Work with your doctor to find the lowest dose that works for you. This helps to avoid potential problems with "brain fog" and withdrawal symptoms that can happen with many drugs prescribed for sleep, anxiety and depression. Discuss any concerns with your doctor or specialist. Do not change doses or stop taking any medication without the guidance of your family doctor or the prescribing doctor. If you just stop taking a medication you are not getting the benefits and your doctor does not have the important information he or she needs to help you manage successfully.

Dental treatment for teeth conditions or jaw pain (temporomandibular or TMJ disorder) can help ease symptoms for many people with tinnitus or sound sensitivity. But dental equipment can be noisy (e.g. drills). Since appointments are short, there is no risk of noise related hearing loss. But the noise can aggravate tinnitus temporarily or be uncomfortable for people with sound sensitivity. If you have concerns, you can use hearing protection during appointments if noisy equipment or drills will be used; some dentists will also allow breaks during drilling to make it easier to cope with (e.g. 5 minutes on, 5 minutes off). Ultrasonic tools used to clean teeth are also very noisy, and have been linked to tinnitus and tinnitus exacerbation in some people. Some dental offices willingly offer alternatives to ultrasonic cleaning devices (e.g. clean teeth using manual tools). Find a dental office where the staff cares about your tinnitus or sound sensitivity needs.

TINNITUS TREATMENT

The focus of this book is non-medical tinnitus treatment usually provided by an audiologist, tinnitus specialist or counselling specialist. Many people also use available treatment approaches to self-manage their tinnitus. Current scientific research is exploring which tinnitus treatment approaches may work best for tinnitus due to specific medical conditions. However, no conclusive data is available yet. There is currently no specific remedy for a specific tinnitus condition. So it doesn't matter what might have caused a person's tinnitus or sound sensitivity. Treatment options are similar for anyone with distress. Treatment options are recommended based on the amount of distress present.

Various tinnitus distress severity categories are currently in use. A simple scheme (not necessarily used by tinnitus specialists) is to use three main categories: slight to mild, moderate, and severe. People with slight to mild severity have tinnitus but aren't particularly distressed by it. People with moderate severity have tinnitus and may be distressed in specific situations (e.g. when it's quiet around them). People with severe severity have tinnitus and are distressed in most daily situations.

For people with slight or mild tinnitus, often no further treatment is necessary. After the tinnitus evaluation and counselling, people usually feel relieved and don't need any further treatment. For mild tinnitus distress, some people will still be motivated to add some coping strategies into their daily life. Formal treatment is not typically needed.

For people with moderate to severe tinnitus distress, some form of treatment is often very helpful. If treatment is recommended, then the care provider and their client should discuss options and explore possible solutions together. The more distressed a person is, the more comprehensive the treatment approach will be. Also the more severe the tinnitus distress, the more likely the person will need formal treatment that includes counselling therapy.

SOUND SENSITIVITY TREATMENT

Sound sensitivity is rare, but if present the distress can be mild, moderate or severe. This book was written for people with tinnitus or tinnitus and sound sensitivity. Much of the information will also apply to people with sound sensitivity alone. Sound sensitivity is reversible through treatment. There are specific ways that tinnitus treatment is modified for people with sound sensitivity. If a person has sound sensitivity and tinnitus, the sound sensitivity is usually treated first. Tinnitus specialists have the knowledge and training on how to adapt treatment for sound sensitivity. Formal treatment from a tinnitus specialist is recommended if you are very distressed by sound sensitivity. Counselling specialists may also be helpful in some cases. Professional help using proven treatment methods is much more beneficial than trying to cope on your own.

Table 4
TREATMENT PLANNING

EVALUATION FINDINGS	TREATMENT OPTIONS
Medical Issue	• Referral to doctor and/or ear specialist
Tinnitus Distress	• Education and reassurance counselling • Sound enrichment • Mind enrichment • Body enrichment • Sleep management
Hearing Loss	• Hearing loss management
Hazardous Noise Exposure	• Hearing protection management
Sound Sensitivity	• Tinnitus treatment (modified) • Hearing protection management (modified)

Education and reassurance counselling was discussed in the chapter on Tinnitus Evaluation. The following chapters describe additional treatment options. Some options are appropriate for everyone (e.g. Body Enrichment, Sleep Management). Some options only apply for certain people, and will need to be customized for their individual needs. For example, anyone with hearing loss will benefit from Hearing Loss Management. Anyone using hearing protection or with concerns about noise exposure will benefit from Hearing Protection Management. Other options will also vary depending on each person and the severity of distress present. For example, Sound Enrichment can vary from environmental sound used as needed to specific ear level devices worn all waking hours. Mind Enrichment can vary from simple distraction techniques used as needed to formal counselling therapy. As a person goes through treatment, the treatment plan will often be updated or adjusted over time. People with tinnitus or sound sensitivity need to work with their care provider to select options and build a treatment plan that is most appropriate for their individual needs.

Author's Case: My severe tinnitus distress started after a car accident. No medical treatment was needed. I have normal hearing. I was a good candidate for tinnitus treatment. I used Sound Enrichment, Mind Enrichment, Body Enrichment, and Sleep Management. Some strategies or tools worked better than others. Over time I have only continued using the tools that have made a noticeable difference in my coping ability. My plan includes tools that I use everyday, as well as additional tools I use for flare-ups. I also use appropriate hearing protection when I have occasional hazardous noise exposure.

Case 20: She was worried that her tinnitus meant she was losing her hearing or had a serious medical condition. Medical evaluation ruled out any problems. Her tinnitus evaluation showed normal hearing and mild tinnitus distress. She received Education and Reassurance. She was interested in Body Enrichment. She did not feel she needed any other specific tinnitus treatment.

Case 21: He reported that he had noticed gradual onset tinnitus in both ears. He was bothered because he felt the tinnitus interfered with conversations. When he saw his family doctor for clearance before starting tinnitus treatment, it was discovered that he had high blood pressure. With appropriate medical treatment, his blood pressure was brought under control. He had a tinnitus evaluation that showed he had hearing loss. He received Education and Reassurance. His tinnitus treatment included Hearing Loss Management.

Case 22: This woman had difficulty with clicking and pain in the jaw (temporomandibular joint or TMJ problem). She worked with her dentist to manage the problem by using special custom fit night guards for her teeth. She found she coped better with her tinnitus when her jaw felt better. She was only disturbed by her tinnitus when she was trying to sleep. Sleep Management was recommended.

Case 23: She reported tinnitus in one ear, imbalance or unsteadiness, and worse hearing in one ear. She was referred to an ear specialist who arranged an MRI of her ears. This test ruled out any underlying medical condition. It was recommended she proceed with further tinnitus treatment. Tinnitus evaluation showed hearing loss, moderate to severe tinnitus distress, and no sound sensitivity. Tinnitus treatment recommendations included Hearing Loss Management, Sound Enrichment, Mind Enrichment, and Sleep Management.

Case 24: He had a hearing loss from working in hazardous noise. He uses hearing protection except when he has to take it off to speak with co-workers. At the end of a workday, he notices his tinnitus is worse. Treatment would focus on Hearing Loss Management and Hearing Protection Management appropriate for both his hearing loss and workplace needs. Sound and Body Enrichment were also recommended.

Case 25: He uses earmuffs for everyday activities including taking the bus and doing his shopping. He is very bothered by his tinnitus and by all the "loud" sounds around him. Formal treatment including Hearing Protection Management is recommended. Treatment would include an appropriate sound desensitization program using sound enrichment, with a plan for decreasing dependence on hearing protection in non-hazardous noise situations. Once sound sensitivity was improved, then tinnitus specific treatment could be started.

HEARING LOSS MANAGEMENT

Blindness separates me from things. Deafness separates me from people. Helen Keller.

Approximately half of the people with tinnitus also have hearing loss. As discussed in the chapter on How We Hear, tinnitus can be present with any type of hearing loss (conductive, sensorineural or mixed). The most common type of hearing loss is a high frequency loss. High frequency hearing loss makes speech sound muffled or unclear. This makes it hard to hear and understand conversations especially when there is background noise around. Straining to hear because of hearing loss can make tinnitus worse.

Many people with tinnitus worry that the presence of tinnitus means their hearing will get worse. Any hearing loss essentially happens independently of tinnitus. If your hearing changes, it is not because of tinnitus. Hearing changes are related to whatever caused your hearing loss. One of the most common types of high frequency hearing loss is age-related hearing loss. People often forget that all humans will experience some hearing changes with age. Typically this starts around age 50 to 60, although age-related hearing loss can appear earlier particularly if other family members had hearing loss as adults. It is important not to blame tinnitus for hearing changes that naturally develop when we get older.

Usually hearing loss creeps up slowly on a person. Other people often notice the hearing loss before the person who has it. Eventually people start to notice hearing difficulties themselves. Many people try to deny the problem, thinking that people today just don't speak as clearly as they used to. Some smile and nod agreeably as conversations slip by them. This can result in mistakes or serious misunderstandings (e.g. but you agreed you would pick me up after dinner).

Case 26: He was at a restaurant with his wife. An old friend who he had not seen in a long time stopped by their table to chat. He had trouble hearing what was said with competing voices from other tables around them. At one point the friend said something and stopped talking. He didn't catch what was said, so he smiled and commented, "That's nice." The friend said good-bye and left abruptly. His wife became very upset and asked what was wrong with him. It turned out his friend had been telling them that his dear wife had just died after a long illness. He decided it was time to find out if he needed hearing aids.

The first sign of hearing loss for many individuals is having a hard time understanding people talking when there are competing background sounds present (e.g. voices, music). Signs of hearing loss include:

- You have trouble hearing in background noise (e.g. at a family dinner, in a restaurant, in the car).

- You have trouble understanding people when they talk from a distance (e.g. from another room).

- You have trouble hearing women's/children's higher pitch voices.

- You know people are talking, but sometimes you can't understand what they say.

- You often ask people to repeat what they say.

- You think many people mumble.

- You strain to hear.

- You bluff and pretend you have heard what was said.

- People accuse you of not listening.

- People complain that you are turning the TV or radio up too loud.

- People walk away from conversations with you because you can't hear them.

Hearing loss and communication breakdowns are difficult to cope with. They can cause frustration, anger, depression and stress. These are all emotional reactions that can also negatively impact on tinnitus. This is particularly true when people don't realize they have a hearing loss that is causing their hearing difficulties. People often blame their tinnitus for their hearing problems. This can make them feel even more frustrated, angry, depressed or distressed over the tinnitus. That is why it is so important for anyone with tinnitus to have their hearing evaluated to see if they have underlying hearing loss. If they do, hearing loss management is an essential tinnitus treatment. Hearing loss management usually includes hearing aids. Communication strategies and additional assistive listening devices can also be helpful. Hearing aids should be obtained through a reputable hearing aid provider, audiologist or tinnitus specialist. Audiologists or tinnitus specialists are the main providers mentioned in this book since they are most commonly involved in tinnitus treatment.

HEARING AID BENEFITS

Hearing aids are devices worn on the ears that analyze and process sound to make it easier to hear for people with hearing loss. Amplification is adjusted or programmed to fit an individual's pattern of hearing loss. Research shows that people with hearing problems often put off getting hearing aids for many years. But the earlier a person is fit with hearing aids, the better their chances are of being successful hearing aid users. There are many reasons why people put off the decision to try hearing aids. They might needlessly worry that other people will judge their appearance or intelligence. People also delay trying hearing aids because they don't recognize the significant impact hearing loss can have on their life. Hearing loss can decrease quality of life by straining relationships, restricting social activities and independence, and jeopardizing safety. Using hearing aids can improve quality of life.

It is obvious that people with moderate or greater hearing loss would be helped by hearing aids. But people with mild hearing loss may not think hearing aids are necessary. People are usually considered borderline or marginal hearing aid candidates when they have only a mild degree of high frequency hearing loss present. A person with slight high frequency hearing loss may only notice occasional difficulties when in background noise. The usual primary goal of hearing aids is to restore hearing and improve communication. A person with borderline hearing loss who does not have tinnitus may wait to get hearing aids since they seldom have communication problems.

However for people with tinnitus, hearing aids don't just restore hearing and improve communication. Hearing aids are also an important component of tinnitus treatment. As discussed in the chapter on How We Hear Tinnitus, tinnitus appears to come from brain over-activity usually associated with silence. With hearing aids there is less silence and more sound. This sound gets processed along the hearing pathways and stimulates nerve fiber networks with sound actually coming from our environment. It is believed using hearing aids can help re-set the brain's hearing system and reduce the over-activity associated with tinnitus.

Hearing aids can also be beneficial for people with tinnitus by providing sound enrichment and mind enrichment. Hearing aids enrich the sound environment by increasing the loudness of sounds around you. More sound from the environment reaches your ears, including sounds that would be missed without the hearing aids. In some cases this can help partially cover up the tinnitus sound. In many cases this can help make the tinnitus seem less noticeable during a person's daily activities. The chapter on Sound Enrichment has additional information on treating tinnitus with sound.

Hearing aids can also help enrich a person's mental state. They can distract or relax a person. Hearing aids distract people's attention towards environmental sounds or voices that are heard more easily through the hearing aids. Hearing aids also reduce the stress of straining to hear. This can help people feel more relaxed which improves overall ability to cope with tinnitus. The chapters on Sound Enrichment and Mind Enrichment have more information on treating tinnitus with distraction and relaxation sound and techniques.

People sometimes wonder whether they should get one hearing aid or two. When a person gets one hearing aid, it is typically called a monaural (one ear) fitting. When a person gets two hearing aids, it is typically called a binaural (both ears) fitting. It is proven that binaural hearing aids worn on each ear give significant benefit (assuming the person has hearing loss in both ears). Reported benefits include better sound quality, better understanding of conversations in background noise, and easier detection of the direction sounds are coming from. Our brain's hearing system is designed to use information coming from two ears. Two hearing aids help keep sound input to the brain as natural as possible.

People who have essentially equal hearing loss in both ears but only wear one hearing aid may gradually lose their ability to understand what people are saying in the unaided ear. Auditory deprivation is the term used to explain this reduced speech understanding in the unaided ear. If we stop exercising our legs, our muscles can lose their ability to function. If we stop "exercising" our ears, the hearing system can lose its ability to process sound. It is still possible to get a second hearing aid after auditory deprivation has happened. But it can take a long time to restore speech understanding and hearing ability. It is important to know that the hearing system does not always recover the speech understanding ability that could have been maintained if someone started off with two hearing aids.

Sometimes people are not a candidate for two hearing aids. They might have an unaidable ear (typically due to medical or hearing loss related reasons). When a person is not a candidate for two hearing aids, they can still benefit from a monaural (one ear) hearing aid fitting for their aidable ear. Other hearing aid technology is also available. For example, some people find benefit from a CROS (Contralateral Routing of Signal) technology hearing aid. This technology takes sound from the person's unaidable ear, and transfers it to the person's better ear to be heard. Cost is also often a factor in whether a person can get one or two hearing aids. However, if you are a candidate for two then it is most beneficial to get two if you can.

HEARING AID STYLES

Hearing aids in general are custom made for the shape of the ear. Behind The Ear (BTE) styles sit behind the ear and have a custom earmold attached that sits in the ear canal opening. Custom made completely in ear hearing aids include In The Ear (ITE) or the smaller In The Canal (ITC). ITE styles sit in the ear canal opening and extend partly into the ear canal. ITC styles sit in the ear canal although the hearing aid can still usually be seen if someone is looking into your ear. The ITD (In The Drawer) style of hearing aid is never used or only used occasionally. It spends most or all of the time sitting in a drawer. The ITD style of hearing aid gives no benefit for hearing loss or tinnitus.

Too many people choose an ITE or ITC hearing aid because they think it is the smallest or the most invisible. Cosmetic appearance or visibility is not an appropriate reason to choose a hearing aid style. The size or style of hearing aid selected should depend on ear canal size, pattern of hearing loss present, and technology features required. Larger style hearing aids have the potential to be more technologically advanced, because the hearing aid manufacturers have more room to fit components and features into the hearing aid. Smaller aids are not necessarily the wrong choice, but their main sales point is usually their size. Small custom in the ear sizes may come with fewer technological features, less power (amplification boost) and often less reliability (more frequent repairs).

With many styles of hearing aids, the ear canal is blocked off either by the hearing aid itself, or by the earmold used to hold the hearing aid in place. When the ear canal is closed or blocked off it is called occlusion. Occlusion is known to make tinnitus seem louder. Stick your fingers in your ears, and it will likely make your tinnitus sound more noticeable. A similar effect can happen when you put hearing aids in your ears. With hearing aid occlusion effect, natural sound appears muffled, a person's voice can sound strange or loud, and tinnitus can seem louder when the hearing aids are worn. This occlusion effect happens when hearing aids are a style that block up a person's ear canals too much. Many people don't like wearing their hearing aids because of the occlusion effect.

To prevent or minimize occlusion, hearing aid styles can be selected that keep the ear canal as naturally open as possible. This is called an open fitting. Open fittings can sometimes be obtained through the use of large airflow vents in more standard styles of hearing aids. With some recent technology open fittings, the hearing aid is a tiny Behind The Ear style, and a thin tube, wire or custom earmold is used to carry sound from the hearing aid to the ear canal. Some manufacturers are now offering similar open fittings in a tiny style that fits in the ear canal. Open fittings are often recommended for people with tinnitus.

Many people with tinnitus find open fittings very comfortable, pleasant, and natural sounding. However, this option may not be appropriate for people with significant low frequency hearing loss, severe or profound hearing loss, or problems with manual dexterity needed to handle and use these tiny hearing aids. Your audiologist or tinnitus specialist can recommend the hearing aid style that is most appropriate for your hearing loss and tinnitus.

HEARING AID TECHNOLOGY

Modern digital hearing aids allow for complex processing of incoming sound. Hearing aids are now like miniature computers that analyze and process sounds to best amplify them for each individual hearing aid wearer. As well as boosting in the appropriate pitch range for a person's hearing loss, hearing aids also boost an appropriate loudness range. The more hearing loss that is present, the more boost that can be provided. The amount of boost or amplification also depends on the loudness of the sound input. In general loud sounds receive the least boost, moderate sounds receive some boost, and the most boost happens for soft sounds that would otherwise be unheard because of the hearing loss.

Hearing aids also come with various standard and optional technology features. Some of the most commonly used features include multiple listening programs, noise reduction, feedback reduction, volume control, and telecoil technology. However, hearing aid technology undergoes constant innovations. It is impossible to provide specific current information when improvements are constantly taking place in the technology available. A brief description of some of these technology features is provided here. This information is intended to give the reader a very basic general overview of some available features. It is not intended to replace the advice and expertise of your audiologist or tinnitus specialist when selecting an appropriate hearing aid.

One popular feature of modern digital hearing aids is multiple listening programs. This offers the wearer different settings or processing programs for different purposes. For example, a person's hearing aid may have three different programs. One program helps them hear comfortably in background noise. A second program helps them hear soft sounds in quiet situations to help enrich their sound environment. A third program might be used for listening to music. Programs can be changed for each listening situation. Depending on the hearing aid, the user might manually change programs (e.g. by pushing on a button, switch or remote control) or the hearing aid may automatically adjust settings as required based on an analysis of the wearer's listening environment.

Most hearing aid manufacturers also offer features that help improve speech understanding in noisy situations. Noise is often defined as unwanted sound. The problem with hearing loss is that the voice we want to hear is often drowned out by other unwanted competing noise from other voices. Imagine you are at a restaurant or family gathering, and you can't hear the person you are talking to because the voices of other people chatting around you interfere. In the past, standard hearing aids came with one microphone. These single microphones picked up sounds from all directions around you equally (omni directional), and provided "surround sound". However, this technology made listening in background noise difficult since all voices and sounds around the person were amplified or boosted similarly. With one microphone, voices get mixed in together with any other unwanted noise in the environment. A common complaint for people wearing hearing aids was they just couldn't hear well in background noise situations since voices from all around them blurred out the voice of the person they wanted to hear.

To help solve this problem, hearing aid manufacturers now offer multiple microphones to allow directional sound capability as an option on many current hearing aids. Usually we face or look towards the person we are most interested in listening to. Multiple microphones work together to reduce sounds coming from behind you or coming from different directions while the sound or voice you are facing is amplified best. For example if you were standing on a sidewalk facing somebody in conversation, this type of technology could help screen out the noise of a car driving by while still amplifying the person's voice so it was heard clearly. Research shows that the most effective hearing aid feature to help people hear speech better in background noise is multiple microphones.

One problem that happens when hearing aids go into "directional" mode is that the wearer can feel like they are listening in a tunnel as sound from the rear and sides is reduced. Current research suggests that some hearing aid wearers prefer the sound quality when one hearing aid is always set to omni directional (surround sound) and the other hearing aid is always set to directional. This allows them to focus in on individual speakers while still maintaining an awareness of their listening environment. This type of setting is not preferred or recommended for everyone. It is important to work closely with your audiologist or tinnitus specialist to find the most appropriate settings for your hearing loss and listening circumstances.

Hearing aid manufacturers also use noise reduction processing in their hearing aids. This feature mainly helps with sound quality and not with speech understanding. Some forms of noise reduction are designed to screen out soft environmental sounds and any internal noise created by the hearing aid's own microphones. This is not always an advantage for people with tinnitus. In a hearing aid program for quiet environments, noise reduction may need to be turned off to help maintain a softly enriched sound environment. In a program for background noise environments, the noise reduction feature can be turned on for greater listening comfort. Again, people should work closely with their audiologist or tinnitus specialist to set hearing aid programs to the most appropriate noise reduction settings and features for their tinnitus.

Improved feedback reduction is another helpful digital feature offered by hearing aid manufacturers. Feedback is a high pitch squeal or whistle made by the hearing aid in various situations (e.g. hearing aid turned up too high and leaking sound gets re-amplified; hearing aid gets too close to something that sets off the whistle). Often the hearing aid user can't hear the feedback themselves because of their hearing loss, and only find out about it if someone points it out. When hearing aids are feeding back, they are not amplifying sound efficiently. Digital hearing aids can identify and process the feedback signal to reduce or cancel it.

When getting hearing aids, people may need to consider whether they should have a manual volume control. Typically digital hearing aids work automatically to set the hearing aid loudness or amplification depending on the volume of incoming sound. This helps eliminate fiddling with the hearing aid to adjust the volume as sound levels around you change during your day. However sometimes people may find the automatically selected volume isn't what they want. Some manufacturers offer a completely manual (user operated) volume control. The disadvantage is that research shows most people don't set their hearing aids to the best volume for their hearing loss. Other hearing aids with automatic volume control may also have a manual override as an available option. With this feature, the hearing aid processing mainly operates automatically. But the user can still adjust the volume softer or louder when necessary. Many hearing aid users will still prefer fully automatic hearing aids. People who are unable to manually adjust their hearing aid's volume (e.g. problems with finger dexterity, stroke, Parkinson's, etc.) are better off with fully automatic volume control and processing.

One relatively inexpensive hearing aid feature to consider is built-in telephone technology called a telecoil or t-coil. It is often difficult for people with hearing loss to hear over the telephone. On compatible phones, a telecoil allows the hearing aid to pick up the electromagnetic voice signal coming through a telephone, and then amplify it through the hearing aid. When the telecoil feature is turned on, the hearing aid microphone is off and will not pick up surrounding room noise. This can be particularly helpful when you need to use a phone in a noisy environment such as a restaurant or shopping mall. Another advantage of the telecoil is that you can turn up the hearing aid volume to hear phone conversations better without risk of feedback (whistling). Hearing aids need to be a sufficient size to fit in a telecoil. People need to be taught how to correctly use the telecoil on their hearing aid by their hearing aid provider.

Another benefit of hearing aids with telecoils is that they can be used in combination with some types of assistive listening devices to hear more easily in difficult listening situations. This type of technology is installed and available to use in various settings including some churches, theaters, courts, auditoriums, schools, businesses, etc. Assistive listening devices are discussed later in this chapter. Your audiologist or tinnitus specialist can determine if a telecoil would be a useful feature to include on your hearing aid.

Cell phones, digital wireless phones, or communication system technology is also available. Since the technology was originally designed for people with normal hearing, these phones or systems may or may not work well in combination with hearing aid technology. Various hearing aid manufacturers now offer products with communication system compatibility. Performance may vary depending on the manufacturer of your cell phone or communication system as well as the specific features available. However, communication system technology and compatibility is rapidly improving for people using hearing aids. For example, some digital hearing aids are compatible with cell phone Bluetooth® technology allowing the hearing aid to pick up sound directly and wirelessly without having to hold the phone up to the ear. Potential need for compatibility with communication systems should be considered when selecting a hearing aid.

Direct audio input (DAI) is another technology option that allows a hearing aid to be directly connected to an external audio source such as a television, telephone, computer, CD player, or most commonly an assistive listening device. Assistive listening devices are discussed later in this chapter. This type of technology gives a good quality audio signal while cutting out background noise. Direct audio input is not available with smaller styles of hearing aids. Potential need for direct audio input should be considered when selecting a hearing aid.

FITTING AND TRIAL PERIOD

In general, people with tinnitus should consider the following when selecting hearing aid styles and technology:

- People with tinnitus and hearing loss (even borderline or mild) would benefit from hearing aids as part of their tinnitus treatment plan.

- Best results will be obtained from two hearing aids (one in each ear) when both ears have hearing loss and are both aidable.

- The style selected should not block off natural sound coming to the ear. People with tinnitus should consider styles that allow for open fittings.

- If your hearing aid has multiple programs, the quiet setting should still allow soft background sound to be heard. This helps provide ongoing enrichment of the environmental soundscape.

- Technology options to help in various listening situations (e.g. telecoil, direct audio input, communication system capability) should be considered as needed.

- Never wear hearing aids around very loud sounds that could be a noise hazard. See the chapter on Hearing Protection Management for further information on noise hazards and hearing protection for people with hearing loss and tinnitus (or sound sensitivity).

In the end, the best hearing aids are ones that will be used. There is no single manufacturer, style or technology that is best for all people with hearing loss and tinnitus. The best hearing aid depends largely on your expectations, your lifestyle, and your specific circumstances. Some people with tinnitus will be able to get their hearing aids from a reputable hearing aid provider. But if you have significant tinnitus distress or sound sensitivity, you would likely have the best results if you get your hearing aids from an audiologist or tinnitus specialist. The audiologist or tinnitus specialist will take your individual circumstances into consideration (e.g. pattern and severity of hearing loss, tinnitus or sound sensitivity needs, individual ear canal shape/size, physical constraints, communication systems used, lifestyle, hobbies, etc.). Based on evaluation findings and information you provide, your audiologist or tinnitus specialist can select and fit the most appropriate hearing aid technology for you.

After hearing aids are selected and fit, the audiologist or tinnitus specialist should make sure the hearing aids feel comfortable and that they are working appropriately. This is done through standardized measurements of the hearing aid on its own, and more importantly by real ear measurements or performance measurements of the hearing aid working in your ear. The size and shape of a person's ear canal can change how a hearing aid will amplify once it is put in the ear. It is essential for your hearing aid provider to check actual hearing aid performance with each hearing aid in your ear to make sure it is amplifying properly for your hearing loss. The hearing aids can be adjusted as needed to maximize performance. The next step is to get used to hearing through the hearing aids.

Most people struggle with hearing loss for many years before seeking help. The brain adjusts to incomplete information coming through the hearing system. People with hearing loss often recognize that they are having difficulty hearing certain sounds or in certain situations. Frequently people don't realize that what they can still hear is not being heard to its full extent. When a person is fit with hearing aids, the hearing aids suddenly bring back all those missing and incomplete sounds. Everything sounds strange and different. This might include the sound of your own voice, water running, the telephone ring, the sound of clothes rustling as you walk, the sound of appliances like the refrigerator or computer, etc. Your brain will not instantly adapt to the new sounds. It takes time and practice for your brain to adapt to hearing and start better processing the sounds coming through the hearing aids.

Acclimatization is an improvement in benefit (usually in speech understanding) following the fitting of hearing aids. Research indicates that it takes approximately 2 to 3 months of wearing hearing aids regularly for acclimatization to happen. Once it happens, people notice that they can understand speech better than when their hearing aids were first fit. Sometimes before acclimatization happens, people stop wearing their new hearing aids or don't wear them regularly because they still can't understand words and they think things sound strange. Other people think it is ok to wear their hearing aids "just when they need them". If you have hearing loss, then you need to wear your hearing aids consistently. That is the only way for your brain to get used to processing a full range of sound again.

Your audiologist or tinnitus specialist should give you specific information on how to get used to wearing hearing aids. Some of the following strategies are commonly recommended. Build up your wearing time with the hearing aids. If you are tired after using the aids after a period of time, take them off. You can always take a break and try them again later. Let the way you feel be your guide. The goal is to build up to full time use. The more you wear your hearing aids, the better your brain will become at interpreting the sounds from the hearing aids. Don't be discouraged by the interference of background sounds. Remember you are learning new habits or relearning old habits in a new setting. You will need to learn to identify various background sounds. You will also learn to discriminate (as your brain learns to differentiate) between background sounds and speech. As your brain adapts, you will get better at ignoring competing sounds just as people with normal hearing do.

Use the hearing aids first in your home environment. You may temporarily be disturbed by background sounds. Once you identify your environmental sounds (e.g. running water, the hum of the fridge, the clinking of dishes) these sounds will be less distracting. Get used to listening to just one person. After some practice, try to understand your companion's conversation with a radio or television on. Try to practice locating the source or sound by listening only. Localization of sounds (the direction where the sound is coming from) often presents a special problem to wearers of hearing aids. One exercise that helps to develop this skill is to relax in a chair, keep your eyes closed and have someone attempt to speak to you from different places in the room. Each time your helper changes position, attempt to locate him or her through the sound of their voice alone.

Practice to learn to discriminate different speech sounds. Prepare a list of words that differ in one sound only (e.g. food/mood, see/she, could/good, etc.). Have your helper pronounce these words slowly and distinctly. Watch the lip movements closely while you carefully listen for the differences in similar pairs of words. Then have your helper cover their mouth and pronounce the words again, while you try to discriminate the words by listening alone. Listen to something read aloud. A good exercise in listening is to have your helper read aloud from a magazine or newspaper while you follow along with your own copy of the reading material.

Gradually increase the number of people you talk with. Try having conversations in small groups (e.g. 3 or 4 people) instead of just one on one. Be aware that any additional background noise (e.g. background music) will make it that much harder to hear. Gradually increase the number of situations where you use your hearing aids. After you have adjusted fairly well in your own home to background sounds and to conversation with several people at once, you will be ready to try your hearing aids at the supermarket, coffee shop, church, theatre, and other public places.

As discussed above, acclimatization to hearing aids usually takes 2 to 3 months. Most manufacturers offer a 2 to 3 month trial period for new hearing aids. Usually the longer the trial period the better to allow sufficient time to notice the benefits of adjustment or acclimatization. The hearing aid wearer also gets a chance to try the hearing aids in their daily life during the trial period. They can then report back on any difficulties or concerns they are having. For people with tinnitus, hearing aids should either have no effect on the tinnitus or give some relief (e.g. by providing additional sound that makes tinnitus less noticeable). For people with significant sound sensitivity, it should be treated first before considering hearing aids. Any concerns with hearing aids should be dealt with in the trial period.

A hearing aid fitting may take several weeks and require multiple visits to the audiologist or tinnitus specialist. Modifications or adjustments to the hearing aid fit or processing are often needed during the trial period to fine-tune the hearing aids further for each person's individual needs. Most clinics will provide "check-ups" as needed during the trial period for modifications or adjustments. Usually the first "check-up" should happen after you've worn the hearing aids for at least a week or more. Best results are obtained when the hearing aid user and the hearing aid provider work together over time. When hearing aids are working well and you have practiced and adjusted to them:

- The earmold or hearing aid should be comfortable.

- The sound of your own voice should be acceptable.

- You should be able to hear average speech at a comfortable level.

- Loud speech should be loud but not uncomfortable.

- In a quiet situation you should hear better with hearing aids than without hearing aids.

- In a background noise situation, you should hear better with hearing aids than without hearing aids.

- With hearing aids, you will not hear as well in background noise as in quiet.

- Hearing aids will not make your hearing as good as you remember it to be.

- Hearing aids will not make your hearing normal again. Hearing aids will help you hear better, but not perfectly.

- Hearing aids should make no apparent difference or provide some relief for your tinnitus.

In the majority of cases, people find hearing aids very beneficial as adjusted during their trial period. But if the hearing aids are still not helpful to you, you should return them to the provider. If necessary, the hearing aid can be exchanged or returned to the manufacturer. Make sure you don't keep your hearing aids past your trial period if you are having difficulties. Returns are not usually accepted after the trial period ends. It is a good idea to get written details on the trial period including the specified time the aids may be returned for a refund or credit and whether any non-refundable charges apply.

HEARING AID CARE

Your audiologist or tinnitus specialist should give you information on how to care for your hearing aids. Hearing aids are delicate electronic devices. They should be "stored" in your ears for the majority of your waking hours. There are only a few circumstances where you should not wear your hearing aids. This includes when you are sleeping, when the aids might get wet (e.g. bathing, showering, swimming) or when the aids might be around excess heat, dust, water or hazardous noise. When they are not in your ears, they should be stored safely, usually in the case they come in. If you have pets or small children around, be especially careful to store your hearing aids in a safe place. The small batteries might look like a candy, but can be very harmful if eaten. If this happens, get immediate emergency medical attention. In addition, hearing aids are strangely attractive to most pets. If they are in reach, pets will try to eat the hearing aids and damage them beyond repair.

> **Case 27:** He left his hearing aids on the table. His cat knocked them off with her paw, and his dog crunched them up off the floor. All that was left were some fragments. Luckily, the batteries weren't eaten.

Hearing aids typically last 5 or more years. If problems come up during a hearing aid's lifetime, the manufacturer can often repair them. It is not unexpected that hearing aids should break down every now and then. The ear canal is a warm, humid environment full of salty earwax. These types of conditions would be harmful to any electronic device. A routine clean and check done as recommended by your hearing aid provider (e.g. once a year) often helps to reduce breakdowns. You should also clean and maintain the hearing aids yourself as recommended by your hearing aid provider.

Hearing aids will not last if they are damaged beyond repair (e.g. crushed or broken). If the hearing aid breaks down after many years, repairs may not be possible depending on availability of components. Hearing aid manufacturers phase out old models and their component parts as new models are brought in. Your audiologist or tinnitus specialist can let you know if aids are repairable or if it is time to consider new replacement hearing aids.

Sometimes hearing aids may need to be replaced after only a few years. A person's health may change so that their current hearing aid is no longer appropriate (e.g. starts to get constant ear infections and can't use current style of hearing aid). In other cases a person's hearing may change (e.g. due to aging or other reasons). Current hearing aids are quite flexible, and can often be adjusted or re-programmed as needed over time. But sometimes a hearing aid can no longer give adequate performance. Your audiologist or tinnitus specialist can adjust hearing aids to meet changing needs or let you know when a new hearing aid is necessary.

COMMUNICATION STRATEGIES

Hearing aids can certainly help improve communication in various listening environments by making it easier to understand speech. However, hearing aids are not always enough especially in difficult listening situations. Communication strategies make it easier to converse by helping people manage better when it is hard to hear. Strategies can include asking the speaker to slow down while talking, watching the speaker's face, turning down or off any background music while talking, etc. Information about specific communication strategies is available through audiologists, tinnitus specialists, books, support groups or formal classes. People with tinnitus and hearing loss can benefit from using communication strategies to help improve speech understanding even better than by hearing aids alone.

ASSISTIVE LISTENING DEVICES

Many hearing aid wearers are not happy with their hearing aid performance in noisy situations even when using communication strategies. Noisy or difficult listening situations can include trying to listen in a car, a restaurant, a meeting, in a class, etc. Assistive listening devices (ALD's) are devices than can be used with hearing aids (if compatible) or alone to help a person hear and understand speech better in difficult listening situations. They are sometimes described as "binoculars for the ears". Many assistive listening devices are specifically aimed at helping in background noise since this is where hearing aids work least well. Hearing aids must have specific built in features to work with assistive listening devices. Often ALD's work through a hearing aid's "direct audio input" feature or through a hearing aid's "telecoil" technology. Potential compatibility with assistive listening devices should always be considered when selecting a hearing aid.

FM Systems are one type of assistive listening device that is very effective for improving speech understanding in background noise. FM (Frequency Modulated) Systems are a technology that uses a separate microphone. Voice signals entering the microphone are sent to a receiver (stand alone or built into a hearing aid). In the past there was often a wire or cord between the microphone and the receiver, but current systems are usually wireless. These systems make the speaker's voice heard clearly at a constant level while any surrounding background noise is minimized. FM Systems make voices sound closer, louder and clearer. Different microphone or microphone settings are available. Some will let you pick up the sound of a speaker from one direction, while some will let you pick up the voices of several people (e.g. sitting around a table). For example, the microphone can be pointed toward someone speaking in a car, placed in the center of a dinner or conference table, clipped on a shirt collar near the mouth of an instructor, etc. Personal FM systems used alone or in combination with hearing aids can be very helpful in various work, school and social situations (e.g. having dinner in a restaurant, going to concerts or church). Hearing aids must be FM compatible to work with FM Systems. People with tinnitus or sound sensitivity who don't like the sound quality of FM Systems may prefer good quality hearing aids plus communication skills practice using an auditory training program (e.g. LACE).

A wide variety of other personal or group devices and systems are also available. Besides speech, assistive listening devices can help with hearing various important sounds (e.g. alarm clock, telephone, television, doorbells, smoke detectors, etc.). Some group systems are installed in public places to work for anyone there who has compatible hearing aids or rented a receiver, although group systems are more common in Europe than in North America. Assistive listening devices can improve communication, safety and quality of life. This improvement can reduce fatigue and stress that in turn helps with tinnitus coping. People with tinnitus and hearing aids who still notice hearing or communication problems should seriously consider assistive listening devices.

Associations or organizations for the hard of hearing often have information and resources available on assistive listening devices. Your audiologist or tinnitus specialist should also be a good resource. Ideally before buying, you should be able to see devices demonstrated to see what is available and if it would be helpful for you.

Author's Case: I have normal hearing. But I often have difficulty understanding conversations while in background noise or when the speaker is at a distance (e.g. talking from another room). This is common for many people with tinnitus who also have "normal hearing". I use communication strategies to hear better (e.g. look at who I am listening to, turn down any competing music or walk to a quieter area to talk, let people know when I've missed what they've said, etc.). I will certainly try hearing aids when they would be helpful for me (e.g. because of hearing changes or because of my tinnitus).

Case 28: He was surprised to discover he had hearing loss. He had always thought his hearing was perfect and it was his tinnitus that was making it hard to hear conversations. He tried hearing aids, and after practicing and using them regularly he noticed an improvement in speech understanding. He didn't pay as much attention to his tinnitus after he realized it wasn't the culprit for his hearing problems. No further treatment was necessary.

Case 29: She had hearing loss and very distressing tinnitus. She wanted the smallest hearing aids possible so nobody would know she was wearing them. She was very upset after getting custom In The Canal style hearing aids because her tinnitus became much louder when wearing them. She returned the hearing aids within the trial period, and went to a different clinic to see an audiologist for a second opinion. She tried an open fit style of hearing aids, and found they helped her hearing and made no difference to her tinnitus. She was able to use these hearing aids comfortably. Her audiologist also recommended Sound Enrichment, Mind Enrichment, Body Enrichment and Sleep Management techniques.

Case 30: He had hearing loss and tinnitus that he noticed when trying to sleep. He got hearing aids for his hearing loss, but had concerns during the trial period. He found certain sounds were too loud, and when he was in quiet environments he could really hear his tinnitus. He went back to his audiologist. They adjusted the hearing aid so that sounds never went above being comfortably loud, and so that soft background sounds could still be heard in the quiet program setting. After the hearing aid settings were fine-tuned, he was satisfied with his hearing and tinnitus perception when wearing the hearing aids. His audiologist also recommended an amplified alarm clock, and Sleep Management techniques.

Case 31: He had hearing loss, tinnitus and sound sensitivity. He thought hearing aids might help, but his audiologist recommended treatment for the sound sensitivity first before treating the hearing loss or tinnitus. Hearing aids were not initially recommended. He was referred to a sound sensitivity specialist for formal counselling and sound therapy. Sound Enrichment ear level devices were recommended. Later on in his treatment program, he ended up phasing in use of hearing aids appropriate for his sound sensitivity, hearing loss and tinnitus.

Case 32: He had hearing loss and tinnitus. He usually worked in an office environment, but sometimes had to go into a hazardously noisy area during his workday. He had a lot of communication demands at work (e.g. meetings, making cell phone calls to customers, etc.). His audiologist recommended hearing aids that would accommodate his hearing loss, tinnitus and communication demands. An assistive listening device that was compatible with his hearing aids was recommended to help during meetings. Hearing Protection Management was also recommended for when he went into hazardous noise.

Case 33: She had hearing loss and tinnitus. After being reassured about her tinnitus, she reported that her main concern was difficulty hearing in social situations (e.g. as a passenger in a car, in a restaurant, etc.). Her audiologist recommended hearing aids and an assistive listening device. She noticed a big improvement in understanding conversations in background noise. Her audiologist offered a course on communication strategies. She and her partner took the classes, and began using and benefiting from various communication strategies. Her audiologist also recommended additional Sound Enrichment techniques.

SOUND ENRICHMENT

Why is it that the buzzing in the ear ceases if one makes a sound? Is it because the greater sound drives out the less? Hippocrates.

JUST DON'T LISTEN TO IT

Everyone has the potential to hear the "sounds of silence". This potential is greater in quiet situations like reading, concentrating, relaxing, or trying to fall or stay asleep. Many people with tinnitus are told, "Just don't listen to it". This is not the most helpful advice unless practical tips on "how not to listen to it" are also provided. One of the best ways to not listen to tinnitus is to listen to something else. That is why all people with bothersome tinnitus should avoid silence. The concept of fighting fire with fire is a useful analogy for tinnitus. You can use other sounds to fight the sound of tinnitus.

It is well established in the scientific literature that the presentation of one sound can change the perceived loudness of a second sound. Tinnitus can reduce in loudness or disappear completely following sound stimulation. As described in the chapter on Tinnitus Evaluation, this effect is called residual inhibition. The effect typically lasts only a few seconds to a few minutes once the outside sound is turned off. Keeping outside sound turned on can maintain the effect. There is no doubt that the regular use of appropriate sound can have a positive long-term effect on tinnitus. Research also shows that people have reduced or improved sound sensitivity through using sound enrichment.

Sound enrichment or sound therapy is the specific use of soft to moderate sound to help make it harder to hear tinnitus during day or night situations. The sounds selected are more pleasant to listen to than tinnitus and may help make it less noticeable or less a focus of attention. Sound enrichment is also used to de-sensitize the hearing system for people who are sensitive to sound. This type of therapy keeps your hearing system busy with sound coming from outside of your body. This is the type of sound your hearing system should be busy with. You can use sound enrichment to take control and actively do something to gain some degree of relief. For many people, this leads to better coping. Remember that two main factors contribute to tinnitus distress:

Sounds of Silence (Tinnitus)

plus Negative Emotional Reaction

equals TINNITUS DISTRESS

Sound enrichment does not get rid of the tinnitus sounds. It uses additional sound to help control the sounds of silence. Sound enrichment can eliminate or reduce how much we can hear the tinnitus over our environment. Some researchers and tinnitus specialists believe that sound enrichment helps decrease the sensitivity of any hyperactive nerve fibers. It may help reset these nerve fibers to become less active and less responsive. This could be helpful for tinnitus and sound sensitivity. The two basic ways of using sound as tinnitus therapy are to use sound as a relaxing background soundscape or to use sound to distract attention from tinnitus. If you have hearing loss, then using hearing aids can help you take full advantage of relaxation or distraction sound enrichment. This chapter also describes sound enrichment for sound sensitivity.

RELAXATION SOUND ENRICHMENT

Sound is commonly used to increase feelings of relaxation. Imagine you go to the spa for a massage. Soothing sounds will often be playing in the background to help improve relaxation. Imagine you go to the dentist for an appointment. Soothing music will generally be playing in the background to help improve relaxation and lower any anxiety, fear or stress. Sound can soothe, calm and comfort.

Having sound in the background can be relaxing because it helps make tinnitus less noticeable. A light in a dark room will look much brighter than the same light in a sunny room. A sound in a quiet room will seem much louder than the same sound in a noisy room. In the same way, tinnitus will seem louder in a quiet environment than in a noisy environment. Consider how much you notice your tinnitus when you are in a busy restaurant compared to when you are sitting at home quietly reading a book. Less noticeable tinnitus is an improvement that helps people cope better.

For many years, people with tinnitus have used relaxing background environmental sounds or music for sound enrichment. Relaxation sound is also often used for sound sensitivity therapy. Your goal is to create a comfortable "sound ambiance" or soundscape. What may be pleasant for one person may be unpleasant for another person. Let the sounds you enjoy help guide you. The key to effective use of relaxation sound is that the sound used should be easily ignored, comfortable and pleasant. There is a huge variety of sounds available including but not limited to white noise, nature sounds, music, or other sounds or sound effects you find helpful.

White Noise is a very helpful sound for most people with tinnitus. It is also helpful for people with sound sensitivity. Just as white light contains all colors, white or wide-band noise contains all tones or frequencies. It typically sounds like a hissing or "shhhhh" type noise. White noise is a good neutral background sound that is easily ignored. The sense of relaxation doesn't just come from the white noise itself. It comes from the effect that white noise has on tinnitus. White noise makes tinnitus less noticeable. This effect can make people feel less tense and more relaxed.

White noise also stimulates a good cross section of nerve fibers as the white noise is processed through our hearing system. It is believed by some researchers that this may help with suppression of any overactive hearing system nerve fibers. Many people have tinnitus that seems to be suppressed most effectively by noise in a frequency range that includes their tinnitus. Since white noise includes all frequencies it is commonly used for tinnitus treatment. Several methods of formal sound therapy for tinnitus or sound sensitivity use white noise in various sound enrichment situations.

Pink noise is also often recommended as a relaxation type sound for sound sensitivity. It contains sound with more energy at lower frequencies which makes it similar to the range of everyday sound. It could be described as white noise minus the higher frequencies. This can make pink noise more comfortable to listen to than white noise for people with sound sensitivity.

Nature Sounds can also be helpful for relaxation sound enrichment. Any soothing sounds from our natural environment can be used. This might include the sounds of moving water (ocean waves, streams, river, waterfall, fountain). Some people prefer bird or animal sounds (e.g. birdsong, crickets). Others may prefer weather sounds (e.g. wind, raindrops, or thunderstorms). Nature sounds are easily accessible by opening a window, sitting outside, or enjoying the outdoors (e.g. walking, hiking, swimming, golfing, skiing, etc.). Garden sounds (e.g. wind chimes, fountains or water features) can provide a pleasant background soundscape. A birdfeeder will attract birds that cheep and sing. Various devices are also available that can play nature sounds.

Music is an easily available form of relaxation sound enrichment. Most people enjoy music. Typically people already own machines or devices that can play music. Music can be used as relaxation sound if it is pleasant and easily ignored. Instrumental music is often useful as relaxing background sound. Any enjoyable music can provide a comfortable, pleasant, relaxing sound environment. Music typically varies in volume, and can have quiet periods between songs that may limit its helpfulness for tinnitus. People with tinnitus should try listening to different types of music to see which is most helpful for them. Some formal sound therapies use specially processed music played through custom devices to treat tinnitus. A special type of relaxing background music called fractal music is created using a mathematical algorithm or calculation. The benefit of fractal music is currently being studied for people with tinnitus.

Specific Sounds or Sound Effects can be helpful for sound enrichment depending on individual preference. For example, some people may find the humming and bubbling sounds from a fish tank soothing. There has been a case reported where the sound of a train whistle was most effective for one person. A helpful relaxing sound for one person may not be comfortable, pleasant or easily ignored by someone else. Consider your own hobbies, likes and dislikes. Find the sounds that help create a comfortable or relaxing soundscape for you.

DISTRACTION SOUND ENRICHMENT

Distraction sound can draw your attention away from your tinnitus. It is hard for people to pay close attention to more than one sound at a time. Imagine you are having a conversation or busy focusing your attention on a particular sound. It becomes harder to pay attention to tinnitus when you are distracted by another sound or voice. Less awareness of tinnitus is an improvement that helps people cope better. The key to effective use of distraction sound is that the sound should be interesting, comfortable and pleasant.

Many of the sound types described for relaxation sound enrichment can also be used as distraction sound. It depends on how the sound is used whether it easily ignored or actively attended to. For example, music can be ignored in the background or listened to more carefully (e.g. memorizing lyrics or singing along to your favourite song). Nature sounds like birdsong may be ignored in the background or listened to carefully if someone is trying to identify specific birds by their chirps or songs. Music is more easily used as a distraction sound than other types of background sounds like white noise or nature sounds. This is especially true of music with singing. There are also other specific distraction sounds available including but not limited to speech signals, conversation, or task related sounds or sound effects.

Speech Signals can be a helpful distraction for people with tinnitus. Possible speech signals can include movies, comedy programs, talk radio or talk shows, news, sports programs, recorded lectures or recorded books. However, it is very important to avoid subjects or topics that cause strong emotions, stress, anxiety or sadness. Distraction sound that causes a negative emotional reaction is not the goal for tinnitus treatment. Interesting, pleasant and funny topics are generally most helpful.

Conversation is a good way of paying attention to other people instead of tinnitus. Talk about topics that don't include tinnitus. Pleasant, funny or interesting conversation will be most successful in keeping your attention.

Task-Related Sounds or Sound Effects can also be used for distraction sound enrichment. Sounds can be work or hobby related. Many jobs require some degree of listening to equipment or people (e.g. truck driver, teacher). Many hobbies involve listening to specific sounds. For example, if you play a musical instrument or dance, then practice or performing will require you to listen. If you take a class or course (e.g. golf, language, yoga, meditation, pottery, photography, etc.), then you will need to focus on the instructor. A helpful distraction sound for one person may not be comfortable, pleasant or interesting for someone else. Consider your own hobbies, likes and dislikes. Find the sounds that work best for distracting you from your tinnitus sound.

Table 5
SUMMARY OF SOUND TYPES

Relaxation	• White noise
Relaxation or Distraction	• Nature or specific sounds or sound effects (e.g. water, birds, animals, weather, hobby, task related) • Music
Distraction	• Speech (e.g. comedy, sports, movies, news, talk radio, TV, recorded book, conversation)

SOUND MACHINES AND DEVICES

Sound is not always available in our environment. People with tinnitus often need to create their own soundscape. Sound generating machines or devices are a helpful option used by many people with tinnitus (or sound sensitivity). These devices can be wearable personal listening devices or can be stand-alone. Stand-alone devices (e.g. sit on a tabletop) are useful in any quiet room where the person with tinnitus spends time. Personal listening devices are worn on the ears and taken along wherever a person goes. Depending on the severity of the tinnitus distress and the treatment approach used, sound machines or devices may be turned on continuously throughout the day and/or night, or just turned on when the person with tinnitus is spending time in a quieter environment.

There are several categories of sound machines and devices that include but are not limited to tabletop sound machines, sound pillows, tinnitus relief compact discs (CDs), audio equipment (e.g. radio, CD, personal listening systems), computers, appliances, and hobby equipment. Wearable devices specifically for tinnitus include hearing aids, in-ear sound generators and combination instruments. These devices are helpful for daytime sound enrichment because they bring sound straight to the ears.

Tabletop Sound Machines are quite widely available through tinnitus or hearing clinics, retail stores or the Internet. These sound machines typically play a variety of relaxing background sounds including nature sounds and white noise.

Some types of formal sound therapy for tinnitus or sound sensitivity include use of tabletop sound machines playing white noise or pink noise. These devices can be helpful for sleep, reading and concentration. Some tabletop sound machines have the capability (input jack) to be used with a sound pillow that some people use for sleep sound enrichment. If selecting a tabletop sound machine, it should have three main features. It should have a variety of sounds including white noise (and/or pink noise capability if needed for sound sensitivity). It should have a volume control. It should not have an automatic shut-off. After being turned on, the machine should be able to run constantly until turned off.

Sound Pillows are accessories sometimes used with tabletop sound machines. They are made up of a small speaker inside a bed pillow. When the sound pillow is plugged into the tabletop sound machine, the sound is played through the pillow speaker. Sound pillows bring the sound enrichment right by the head instead of the sound enrichment being a backdrop in the room. The idea is that whoever is lying on the pillow hears the sound enrichment, and nobody else in the room is bothered by the sound. These devices are mainly available through tinnitus specialists, hearing clinics or the Internet. Some people find sound pillows very helpful. Typically only one style of pillow is available, which may not be comfortable for everyone. When breakdowns occur, sound pillows are not usually repairable. Sometimes people make their own sound pillow by getting a flat speaker (e.g. from an audio equipment store) to use inside their regular pillow. Some people prefer not to use a sound pillow because their tabletop sound machine used alone gives the side benefit of helping to cover up any other noises in the bedroom (e.g. snoring).

Tinnitus Relief CDs are specifically designed for people with tinnitus. These CDs are currently available through Petroff Audio Technologies and the Oregon Health Sciences University (Oregon Hearing Research Center). The Petroff Dynamic Tinnitus Mitigation™ CDs have specially engineered noise formats including air, water and nature sounds alone or in combination with relaxation sounds and music. The Oregon Health Sciences University Moses-Lang CD has 7 types of specially engineered noises. Some people with tinnitus find the noise tracks closest to their own tinnitus sound are the most helpful to use.

Various researchers and clinics are also exploring the use of custom CDs using sounds or noise burned to a CD that closely matches the person's own tinnitus pitch and loudness as determined through tinnitus evaluation testing. These custom CDs are typically much more expensive than other available

CDs. While some people are helped by sounds resembling their tinnitus, other people are helped by very different sounds. For example, there have been cases reported of low pitch sound used to give relief to a person with high pitch tinnitus. Expensive individualized tinnitus specific custom CDs should be viewed cautiously until more research data on effectiveness is available.

Audio Equipment is an easily available option for relaxation or distraction sound enrichment. Tabletop or wearable radios, CD, or personal listening systems can be used. A huge variety of sounds are available from music, nature sounds, white noise, pink noise, or other sound effects. Some radios or alarm clocks have built-in background nature sounds. Some people use their radio tuned to static between stations, although a white noise device is often preferred since many people find static sounds annoying. Alarm clocks, radios and TVs can also be used for various distraction sound enrichment including news, talk shows or sports programs. Personal listening systems that are portable and wearable are helpful in providing sound in various situations. If you have hearing loss, compatible hearing aids can now link directly and wirelessly to some personal listening systems. Personal listening systems can be hazardously noisy if turned to higher volume. Care should be taken to keep the volume at only a soft to moderate loudness (e.g. half volume or lower).

Computers can be used for sound enrichment. Computers can play a wide assortment of music or sounds from various sources. Internet shows and clips can be played on the computer for distraction sound. Computer software is available which includes various relaxing sounds (e.g. nature, white noise, pink noise, sound effects) to play on the computer at home or at work. Computers can also be used to search out sound files on the Internet. Some people use their computer to set up helpful sounds or sound effects files that they can then play on their personal listening system. It is also possible to use a computer to take a short track of helpful sound or noise (e.g. a few minutes long) and convert it into a longer playing track. The longer track can be played through a personal listening system on repeat mode for more continuous sound enrichment. Computer security precautions should always be taken before downloading any information, data or software from the Internet or other sources.

Appliances can be used for sound enrichment. Fans, air conditioners and air purifiers can all provide reasonable white type noise as a backdrop. These devices may have different settings (e.g. low or high) that also change sound loudness.

But they don't have the ability to adjust the volume in small steps like some other devices. If the sound quality and sound loudness produced by an appliance is comfortable and not annoying, then it can possibly be a suitable device option.

Hobby Equipment sound is often helpful for sound enrichment. This can vary greatly depending on people's personal interests (e.g. musical instruments, fish tanks, bird feeders, garden features). Fountains typically provide a soothing relaxing water sound effect. Small tabletop indoor fountains are now available, although make sure to protect tabletops from water splashes. Many outdoor water features (e.g. stand alone fountains) are offered through various stores and garden centers. Distraction sound sources might include hobby tools or equipment (e.g. woodworking, car repair) although proper hearing protection should always be used whenever loud sound is present.

Hearing Aids are the most recommended type of wearable device for people with hearing loss and tinnitus. As discussed in the chapter on Hearing Loss Management, hearing aids help restore hearing and reduce straining to hear which is always beneficial for tinnitus. Hearing aids also provide sound enrichment by boosting relaxation or distraction sounds around you. Some hearing aids can even play other types of sound (e.g. music) on certain program settings. If a person is a hearing aid candidate, then hearing aids are usually the first step in tinnitus treatment. In some cases, no additional treatment is needed other than hearing aids and tinnitus counselling (education and reassurance). Ideally, hearing aids should be obtained from an audiologist or tinnitus specialist.

In-Ear Sound Generators are sometimes helpful for people with tinnitus and/ or sound sensitivity who have normal hearing. In-ear sound generators are mini sound machines that play white noise. In-ear sound generators look similar to a hearing aid, and are worn during the day in the ears. The noise volume can be controlled in small, precise steps. An advantage of these devices is that the white noise is available continuously during the day. Sound enrichment is always available at the ears. These devices can be helpful for people with sound sensitivity since the noise is easily set to a preferred comfortable loudness. These devices are expensive so cost can be a factor. In-ear sound generators are most commonly recommended as part of formal sound therapy. They are typically used continuously during initial treatment, and may be gradually phased out (and only used as needed for flare-ups) once sound sensitivity or tinnitus coping has improved. They should only be obtained and used under the guidance of an audiologist or tinnitus specialist.

Combination Instruments are also helpful for some people with hearing loss as well as tinnitus and/or sound sensitivity. They are wearable in-ear devices that combine a hearing aid and an in-ear sound generator. They are worn during the day in the ears. The hearing aid technology available in a combination instrument often has a poorer quality signal or more limited features than available on stand-alone digital hearing aids. Multiple controls for the hearing aid and sound generator may be difficult to manage for some people. These devices are expensive so cost can be a factor. Combination devices are most commonly recommended as part of formal sound therapy. Amplification and sound enrichment is always available at the ears. For people with sound sensitivity, usually only the white noise component is used at first to treat the sound sensitivity and then the hearing aid component is introduced later in the treatment process. Combination devices are typically used continuously during initial treatment, and may be replaced with hearing aids (with the combination devices available to be used as needed for flare-ups) once sound sensitivity or tinnitus coping has improved. They should only be obtained and used under the guidance of an audiologist or tinnitus specialist.

Many people with tinnitus don't like in-ear sound generators and combination instruments. Some people prefer other sound types instead of constant white noise for daytime use. Some people feel they have enough noise from their tinnitus, and they don't want extra white noise from these devices right in their ears. Some people prefer the better technology of a stand-alone hearing aid that can be used with sound enrichment from other devices in their environment. In general, in-ear sound generators and combination instruments have been found most helpful in combination with counselling therapy for people with severe sound sensitivity or severe tinnitus distress. Because these devices are not appropriate for everyone with tinnitus, they should only be obtained from an audiologist or tinnitus specialist who has determined if you are a candidate for this type of device. The device should be returned within the trial period if unsuccessful.

Table 6
SUMMARY OF SOUND MACHINES OR DEVICES
(In addition to hearing aids)

White Noise	• Available devices (that can also be used for pink noise if capable) include tabletop sound machine (sound pillow optional), audio equipment, computer, in-ear sound generator, combination instrument, etc. Other white noise type devices include fan, air conditioner, air purifier, etc.
Nature or Specific Sounds	• Available devices include tabletop sound machine, audio equipment, alarm clock with nature sounds, computer, fish tank, garden sounds from wind chimes, birds at birdfeeder, fountain or water feature, hobby or task sounds, etc.
Music	• Available devices include audio equipment, radio, computer, TV, musical instruments, custom music devices, etc.
Speech	• Available devices include TV, radio, audio equipment, computer, people, etc.

FORMAL SOUND THERAPY

Formal tinnitus treatment approaches all recommend that people establish a continuous background of soft to moderate sound using various devices. Hearing aids are a key component of tinnitus treatment if hearing loss is present. Tabletop sound machines playing white noise may be used for daytime or sleep sound enrichment. In-ear sound generators (white noise) or combination instruments (white noise plus hearing aid) are sometimes used for sound therapy as part of formal treatment. Music devices with customized processing are also used in some treatment approaches.

The purpose of sound enrichment is to increase the amount of sound a person is exposed to. The loudness level selected or amount of sound recommended depends on the treatment approach being used. The term "masking" is sometimes used to describe the effect of covering up the sound of tinnitus with another sound. At a non-masking loudness level, the outside sound and tinnitus can both be heard clearly. As the loudness of the outside sound is increased, eventually the tinnitus and the outside sound will start mixing or blending together without changing or masking the tinnitus sound. As the loudness continues to increase, partial masking can begin to happen. With partial masking, the tinnitus and outside sound blend together and the tinnitus starts to change (e.g. sound softer or different). As the loudness of the outside sound increases more, some people's tinnitus can be completely masked or covered up to the point that they can't hear their tinnitus any more.

Table 7
AMOUNT OF SOUND ENRICHMENT

Non-Masking	• Both outside sound and tinnitus can be heard clearly. • Outside sound does not mask or cover up tinnitus.
Non-Masking Mixing	• The loudness at the upper range of non-masking. • Outside sound and tinnitus are at a loudness level where the tinnitus sound and the outside sound start to mix or blend together. • Outside sound does not change or cover up tinnitus.
Partial Masking	• The loudness range above non-masking mixing. • Outside sound blends with the tinnitus and changes the tinnitus sound in some way without covering it up. • The tinnitus may sound quieter or different in some way.
Complete Masking	• The loudness range above partial masking. • Outside sound completely covers up the tinnitus. • Tinnitus can't be heard at all.

If you are in formal tinnitus therapy, then you must follow the recommendations of your care provider in setting the loudness of your sound enrichment. The most common formal treatment approaches currently in use are Tinnitus Masking Therapy, Tinnitus Retraining Therapy, Tinnitus Music Therapy, and Progressive Tinnitus Management. These all have good success rates. While these methods each work for some people, there is currently no method that works for everyone.

Tinnitus Masking Therapy was introduced in the 1970s and 1980s. The approach has changed slightly over the years, and is now sometimes called Sound Based Relief. Audiologists or tinnitus specialists may offer this type of sound therapy. Masking therapy uses white noise set to partial or complete masking. The sound therapy is used at a loudness where the tinnitus is either changed or covered up by the outside sound. Tabletop sound machines, in-ear sound generators or combination instruments may be used. The goal of sound therapy is to provide tinnitus relief. There is some counselling, but sound is the primary treatment. Research indicates that approximately 75% of people have tinnitus relief from their masking devices set to partial or complete masking loudness. Some people are not able to partially or completely mask their tinnitus, either because of the loudness of their tinnitus or because the noise becomes too loud or uncomfortable before they get any masking effect.

Tinnitus Retraining Therapy (TRT) was introduced in the 1990s. Only specially trained providers can offer this type of therapy. It is most commonly available through audiologists or tinnitus specialists. The term masking is not used in Tinnitus Retraining Therapy. Tinnitus Retraining Therapy describes the effect of sound therapy as suppression of neural activity. TRT uses white noise set to "mixing" level. Sound therapy loudness is used at or softer than the point where the tinnitus mixes or blends with the outside sound but is not changed in any way. Tabletop sound machines, in-ear sound generators or combination instruments may be used. This sound therapy helps people stop paying attention to their tinnitus. The two primary components of this treatment are the sound therapy and regular directive counselling sessions. Directive counselling is discussed in the chapter on Mind Enrichment.

The overall goal of TRT is for people to habituate to their tinnitus. Habituation is when the person is no longer aware of their tinnitus, except when they focus their attention on it, and even then the tinnitus is not annoying or bothersome. TRT uses a very structured approach with strict sound enrichment requirements (typically 24 hour a day initially). It usually takes approximately 6 to 24 months to complete treatment. Research data indicates up to 80% of people are helped by TRT with devices set at or below mixing loudness. A modified form of TRT sometimes called Auditory Retraining Therapy has also been found very effective to treat sound sensitivity. Some people have difficulty complying with the extended timeframe and rigid requirements of TRT.

Tinnitus Music Therapy that uses customized music to treat tinnitus was introduced in the 2000's. Various forms of music therapy have been used. One that has been reported as effective in recent years is Neuromonics Tinnitus Treatment. This treatment is only available through specially trained providers. It is most commonly available through audiologists or tinnitus specialists. Neuromonics Tinnitus Treatment uses relaxation music specially processed based on the individual person's hearing status and tinnitus characteristics. Because the music is customized, it can be effectively used to mask tinnitus perception at a low comfortable listening level. This is often not possible to do with regular music, especially if a person has hearing loss and tinnitus. The music is listened to through a custom personal sound player with earphones. People use the music at key distress times (usually for at least 2 hours per day to start).

Neuromonics Tinnitus Treatment typically takes 6 months to complete. Research suggests that 80 to 90% of people have significant tinnitus improvement with Neuromonics. People often choose this type of music-based treatment because it is a relatively short treatment program that is reported as effective and pleasant to use. The devices are expensive. This type of therapy is being explored as a potential option for people with sound sensitivity.

Progressive Tinnitus Management (PTM) was formally introduced in 2005. It is available through audiologists. Audiologists have long been involved in providing hearing aids, tinnitus devices and counselling. These professionals use systematic PTM evaluation and treatment methods over time to help guide people to cope better with tinnitus or sound sensitivity. People may use a step by step *How To Manage Your Tinnitus* workbook. PTM is called progressive because treatment is only provided at the level needed depending on how distressed a person is. The PTM sound therapy uses various sound types and devices as appropriate for the individual person. PTM uses sound set to non-masking, partial, or complete masking depending on what best meets the person's needs. The sound enrichment plan may change as the person's needs change over time.

Counselling is also provided. Guidance on how to manage may be done one-on-one or in group education sessions. Psychologists may help with group education or additional counselling therapy. People may prefer a PTM approach since it doesn't usually involve the wait lists and time or travel commitments often involved for other specialized tinnitus treatment approaches. Audiology clinics are widely available, and people should be able to obtain a PTM style approach through the audiologist involved in their tinnitus or sound sensitivity evaluation or in their hearing loss care. The PTM workbook materials can also be used by people who prefer an independent self-help approach.

Table 8
SOUND THERAPY LOUDNESS OPTIONS

Tinnitus Retraining Therapy	• Non-Masking • Non-Masking—Mixing
Tinnitus Masking Therapy	• Partial Masking • Complete Masking
Tinnitus Music Therapy	• Non-Masking • Non-Masking—Mixing • Partial Masking • Complete Masking
Progressive Tinnitus Management	• Non-Masking • Non-Masking—Mixing • Partial Masking • Complete Masking

SLEEP SOUND ENRICHMENT

Additional techniques to help with sleep are discussed in the chapter on Sleep Management. Sleep is often a particular problem for people with tinnitus since the bedroom at night is typically the quietest portion of any 24-hour period. Tinnitus is often most noticeable or loud when a person is trying to fall asleep. This can be a concern at bedtime or if people wake up in the middle of the night. It is often hard to get to sleep or get back to sleep while listening to tinnitus.

Using sleep sound can help people sleep more soundly. Sound enrichment in the background is very helpful for sleep. Getting a good night's sleep can greatly help people cope better with tinnitus.

Any sound type can be used for sleep, although relaxation sound is most often used. The steady sound of white noise helps create a neutral soundscape. Some people enjoy other sounds (e.g. nature, music, audiobook) although sound should be selected carefully to be steady, monotonous and relaxing. Certain people with sound sensitivity may use pink noise. The sound should be set to run constantly throughout the night until you wake up. Sound enrichment should also be used regularly every night for best results.

The sound can be set to whichever level is most helpful (non-masking, mixing, partial masking or complete masking) or as recommended by your care provider. If you start to use sound enrichment for sleep and it seems to make your tinnitus worse, then set the loudness to a softer level. The level can always be gradually increased over time as your ears get used to their nightly "sound massage".

Tabletop sound machines are helpful to use for sleep sound enrichment. Some of these machines can be used with a plug-in pillow speaker (sound pillow) for sleeping so nobody else can hear the sound. Tabletop sound machines should have a volume control so the sound can be set to the most comfortable loudness for you. TV is not recommended as background sound for sleep since the loudness levels can fluctuate widely. However, some people like to use distraction sound to fall asleep (e.g. TV or radio with automatic shut off) with another sound like white noise set to run continuously in the background.

Some people like being able to use one appliance for multiple purposes. For this reason, they might choose an air conditioner or fan for sleep sound enrichment if the sound is acceptable. Fans can be used to cool a room in addition to adding sound to the environment. Air purifiers can also add sound to a bedroom, and have the added benefit of helping clean the air. This can improve breathing, which can lead to better sleep overall. People with allergies, asthma, or snoring issues who find the sound of an air purifier acceptable might consider this option. However, there is no way to specifically adjust the volume of these devices, and filters must be changed or cleaned as directed by the manufacturer to maximize effectiveness. If required, replacement filters can be expensive.

SOUND ENRICHMENT PLAN

If you are in formal tinnitus treatment, then your care provider will work with you to develop a sound therapy plan for your tinnitus or sound sensitivity. People with severe tinnitus or sound sensitivity are encouraged to use sound enrichment under the guidance of a trained care provider (e.g. audiologist or tinnitus specialist). Typically if sound sensitivity is present, then it is treated first. Once a person is coping better with sound sensitivity, then treatment for tinnitus and any hearing loss can be addressed. See the chapters on Mind Enrichment and Hearing Protection Management for more information on the treatment of sound sensitivity.

Many people enrich their sound environment without going to formal therapy. A sound enrichment plan can be helpful. Whether you are in formal treatment or not, a sound enrichment plan should take various factors into consideration. These factors include sound type, sound device, sound loudness, and sound duration. The success of the plan will then rest on your motivation to use sound enrichment.

Sound Type is an important factor to consider. Research has compared various sound types, and some sound types work better for some people than for others. But there is no one sound type that works best for everyone. White noise is the most commonly helpful relaxation sound to use for tinnitus or sound sensitivity. Some experts recommend pink noise for people with sound sensitivity since it matches the frequency range of regular daily sound, and may help improve sound tolerance for everyday sounds.

Other relaxation or distraction sounds such as music, nature sounds, specific sounds (e.g. task or hobby related), and speech signals may also help depending on the person and their daily activities. Most people will likely find it helpful to select specific sound types to use in their specific sound situations. For example, one person might like to listen to music while they sit and read, and white noise while they are sleeping. Another person might use nature sounds during the day and music at night. Find sounds that you are comfortable using regularly and consistently. Using different sound types for different situations is an effective approach for most people with tinnitus.

Sound Device should be selected based on what sound you need played through it. In most cases, the sound is more important than the particular device. In formal treatment, specific wearable ear-level devices (e.g. hearing aids, in-ear sound generators or combination instruments) will often be recommended. Other specific devices (e.g. custom music players, tabletop sound machines) that provide an enriched sound environment may also be used for formal therapy as recommended by the care provider. Formal therapy brings sound to your ears as well as building up sound in the space around you.

Outside of formal therapy, the focus is on building up sound in the space around you so you always have something else to hear besides the tinnitus. People with tinnitus may get hearing aids outside of formal treatment to better cope with their hearing loss. They may enjoy the side benefit of sound enrichment heard through their hearing aids. Outside of formal treatment, many people with tinnitus also use other sound devices to build up their sound environment (tabletop sound machines, radio, TV, personal listening devices, etc.).

There is no one device that works best for everyone in all situations. It is important to identify sound situations where you need sound enrichment (e.g. concentrating, relaxing, etc.). You can then select the device that plays the type or types of sound that best suits your needs. Most people with tinnitus end up with a variety of different devices that they use at different times. The goal is finding and using the devices that work best for you.

Sound Loudness can be set at any level from non-masking to complete masking. It is important to remember that sound enrichment always uses soft to moderate sound. More moderate loudness levels may be helpful for distraction sound while softer sound may be helpful for relaxation sound. Loud sound is never used for sound enrichment. In general, there is no particular soft or moderate loudness for sound enrichment that works best for everyone. The actual loudness level selected depends on the individual person.

Because white noise is a steady continuous sound, it is easier to set the loudness level anywhere from non-masking to complete masking. Many sound types (e.g. nature sounds, music, speech signals, etc.) will naturally fluctuate in loudness so it can be difficult to find a specific masking loudness. If this is the case, then a comfortable, pleasant overall listening level is generally the best option. It is important not to fiddle with the volume, as this tends to focus attention on your tinnitus. Set the loudness to where it is comfortable for you, and then forget about it.

If sound sensitivity is an issue, you will likely only be able to tolerate a minimum amount of sound. People with sound sensitivity not only prefer quiet, but before treatment they also try to lower or get rid of any sound sources around them, even sounds that nobody else finds uncomfortable. This is counter-productive to sound enrichment since it leaves a person without natural ordinary sound to listen to. For sound sensitivity treatment, sound is added to the person's environment very gradually. People with sound sensitivity should set their sound therapy loudness as directed by their care provider.

People with tinnitus often have strong likes and dislikes in terms of how much sound they want to use. The goal is to find the loudness where you get the greatest sense of relief regardless of how much you can hear your tinnitus. The loudness level should be acceptable to listen to for long periods of time. If the loudness is annoying, it is better to reduce the loudness than turn off the sound enrichment. Loudness levels will also likely change over time as the sound enrichment needs change through treatment.

The initial use of sound can often cause increases or changes in the tinnitus sound. This is a normal natural phenomenon that suggests the hearing system is responding to sound therapy. Some people with tinnitus or sound sensitivity will only be able to tolerate a small amount of sound. They may just be able to turn on a sound machine or device, and that is all they can take. This is a totally acceptable use of initial sound therapy. Some sound, no matter how faint, is better than no sound. The sound level can always be gradually increased over a period of weeks or months. Over time, the sound level may be maintained at the increased level.

Other people may find the most relief by starting their initial sound enrichment with complete or partial masking. Complete masking usually works best for people who have tinnitus that is easily covered up. The use of partial or complete masking to change tinnitus (e.g. reduce the loudness or cover it up) can provide a needed sense of control. Over time, the sound level can always be reduced as comfortable to maintain a continuous background of non-masking sound for ongoing tinnitus management.

In general, people should experiment with loudness in different situations. Loudness may vary depending on the sound type, device, and when the sound is used. For example, one person may find the most relief with daytime relaxation sound set to non-masking or mixing loudness, and sleep sound enrichment set to complete masking. Another person may find the most relief from daytime and sleep sound enrichment all set to partial masking loudness. Over the course of using sound enrichment, people may often change the loudness from what they could use when starting treatment to a different volume they can use over time once they are managing better. Sound enrichment may also vary depending on flare-ups. For example, a person may use more sound on a distressing day, and less sound on a better day. The goal is finding and using the amount of sound that works best for you over time.

Sound Duration or how long a person uses sound enrichment on a daily basis certainly affects treatment results. There is some debate over whether sound enrichment should be used 24 hours a day or only when a person is distressed. Formal treatment approaches vary from recommending use of sound from at least 2 hours a day up to 24 hours a day. Some experts recommend at least 6 hours per day of sound enrichment at least to start. Some people break up their sound enrichment into shorter chunks (e.g. 2 hours for 3 times a day). Often a person may use sound for longer timeframes at the start of treatment and later on use sound less (e.g. as needed) for ongoing tinnitus or sound sensitivity control.

Because people often spend at least 6 hours a day sleeping (or trying to sleep), then using sound therapy over that timeframe can be an excellent way to add to your overall hours of daily sound therapy. In general, the length of time a person uses sound enrichment daily likely will vary depending on their individual needs. The more severe the tinnitus or sound sensitivity, then the longer you use sound each day the better. Make sure you use your sound therapy every day for best results. Don't expect overnight results. Sound therapy takes time to have a beneficial effect (often from three to six months).

Using sound enrichment regularly may seem overwhelming, especially to those people with tinnitus or sound sensitivity who prefer quiet. But relaxation and distraction sound enrichment can definitely help people with tinnitus or sound sensitivity. Take control by using sound enrichment. It can definitely help improve coping. When using sound enrichment, consider the following guidelines:

- Use sound enrichment continuously and consistently.
- Choose pleasant, comfortable relaxation sounds.
- Choose pleasant, interesting distraction sounds.
- Use soft to moderate sound.
- Use a loudness that provides the greatest sense of relief regardless of whether you can still hear your tinnitus or not.
- Never use loud sound. The sound level should always be comfortable.

- Set and forget the sound level. Choose a comfortable non-annoying loudness and leave it. It is best not to fiddle with the volume.

- Choose devices that you will regularly use and/or wear.

- Choose devices that fit your budget and lifestyle.

- If sound enrichment makes your tinnitus seem worse, then lower the volume to a softer loudness. Some sound is better than no sound.

- It will typically take up to 3 to 6 months of regular consistent sound enrichment for any benefit to become noticeable (e.g. improved coping).

- Very loud sound can be hazardous to hearing (e.g. chainsaws, power tools, loud music). Use hearing protection when around loud noise or music. See chapter on Hearing Protection Management for information on noise hazards and hearing protection appropriate for people with tinnitus or sound sensitivity.

Sound enrichment is most effective when any negative emotional reaction is also treated. All formal treatment approaches include some counselling along with sound enrichment. In milder cases of distress, counselling may just involve basic education and reassurance. In cases of greater distress, specific counselling therapy or mind enrichment techniques may be appropriate. See chapter on Mind Enrichment for more information.

Author's Case: I have normal hearing and had severe tinnitus distress. But I am one of those people who prefer quiet. I am embarrassed to say it was hard to become motivated to use sound enrichment. After seeing the benefit reported in the scientific literature and seeing so many clients improve after using sound therapy, I finally began to use sound enrichment myself. I began with daytime sound enrichment. At home I used music, TV, and fish tanks for indoor relaxation and distraction sound. For anything with a volume control, I listened at a comfortable loudness although often my husband pushed me to listen slightly louder than I preferred. I had wind chimes, water fountains, and nature sounds (e.g. from birds) for outdoor relaxation sound.

At work I am either in a quiet testing area with soundproof booth or in an office environment. I couldn't bring extra sound into the testing area. In my office, I listened to tinnitus relief CDs played at a comfortable loudness on my computer as long as possible before the sound became annoying. For me, this worked out to approximately 15 minutes at a time for a few hours a day in total. I also had a computer software program installed that plays relaxation nature sounds. Sometimes I would just play music through my computer. Daytime sound enrichment made my tinnitus less noticeable. Over time I also heard my tinnitus perception shift to a slightly softer lower pitch sound especially after using the tinnitus relief CDs regularly.

For a long time I did not use sound enrichment for sleep. Then my asthma specialist recommended I use an air purifier in the bedroom to help my breathing. The air purifier I selected makes a white noise type sound and has two loudness settings. The first night I used it, I slept better since it helped cover up my partner's snoring. But I also noticed my tinnitus didn't stand out as much. I have used this air purifier every night for several years. I set it on the louder setting on nights my tinnitus is more noticeable. Over time, my tinnitus loudness settled down so much that most nights I couldn't hear it over the sound of the air purifier. The only time I don't use the air purifier is when I am sleeping away from home. I substitute a different sound device if possible (e.g. air conditioner or fan). Otherwise I don't worry about it, and just sleep as best I can. I do notice that my tinnitus loudness starts to increase again when I don't use sound enrichment at night.

I no longer use sound enrichment 24 hours a day. With rare exceptions (e.g. on vacation) I always use it for sleep. During the day, it is quietest at work so I always use sound there. Because of the improved air quality and because I like the sound so much, I have an air purifier in my office. It has 6 settings so I have more control over the sound loudness. I set it louder on days my tinnitus is more noticeable. I now use this white noise type sound enrichment for approximately 6 hours a day when I am at work. Sometimes I also listen to music through my computer. At home, I continue to use relaxation and distraction sounds when my tinnitus is noticeable. TV and music now cover up my tinnitus, although when I started with sound enrichment my tinnitus screamed over sounds around me. Keep in mind that tinnitus treatment needs to be planned for each person's individual needs.

Case 34: She had severe hearing loss and tinnitus distress. She was referred for Progressive Tinnitus Management. She obtained hearing aids and a tabletop sound machine for sleep through her PTM provider. She also attended PTM group education sessions on how to manage her tinnitus. The support from others in the group was very helpful. As time passed, she began to cope much better.

Case 35: He had hearing loss and mild tinnitus distress. He noticed his tinnitus during the day, but it didn't affect his sleep. He obtained hearing aids, and used music and nature sounds for daytime relaxation and distraction sound enrichment. He noticed his tinnitus less and coped better with an increased soundscape around him.

Case 36: He had mild hearing loss and moderate tinnitus distress. He found a clinic offering Neuromonics Tinnitus Treatment. After a few months of using this tinnitus music therapy, he noticed significant improvement in his tinnitus.

Case 37: She had hearing loss, tinnitus and sound sensitivity. She attended Tinnitus Retraining Therapy modified for her sound sensitivity needs. She received in-depth counselling and combination instruments. The instruments were originally set for her sound sensitivity needs. As her sound sensitivity improved over the course of treatment, the instruments were adjusted for her tinnitus needs. Eventually she was fit with hearing aids appropriate for her tinnitus. She used the hearing aids most of the time, but switched to the combination instruments if she had a flare up. She had significant improvement in sound sensitivity and tinnitus with treatment.

Case 38: He did not notice tinnitus during the day, but heard it when he was trying to fall asleep at night. He thought it would help him stop hearing the tinnitus sounds, so he began to use earplugs for sleeping. Over time, he began to notice new louder ear sounds. He saw an audiologist who strongly encouraged him to stop using earplugs at night for sleep. He was motivated to try white noise at night. He already had a fan at home. He started using this every night to create a white type noise in his bedroom. Over time, his tinnitus settled down, and he noticed significant improvement in his sleep. He was considering getting a white noise tabletop sound machine for year round use including when it might be too cool to want a fan running in the bedroom.

Case 39: He had normal hearing and reported tinnitus distress during the day and when trying to fall asleep. He was not interested in attending formal sound or counselling therapy. The audiologist recommended day and night sound enrichment. Preferred music, nature and TV sounds were recommended for daytime relaxation and distraction, and a white noise tabletop sound machine was recommended for sleep. It was recommended he add sound into his environment everyday in situations when his tinnitus was noticeable.

At his one month check-up, he reported that he didn't like adding in extra sound. He had tried the white noise at night a few times, but didn't think it made any difference. His audiologist explained that it took time for sound therapy to take effect. It was again recommended that he use sound every day and night consistently to see any benefit. At his next check-up, he reported that he had stopped using sound enrichment. He had no improvement in his tinnitus distress. It was recommended he consider sound enrichment again in future if he became motivated to use it.

Case 40: He had severe hearing loss and tinnitus distress. He received tinnitus counselling and available treatment options were reviewed. He would have to travel approximately 2 hours to get to the nearest Tinnitus Retraining Therapy provider. He decided he would like to try TRT, and was placed on a three month waiting list. Because he was so distressed, he decided to go ahead with hearing aids for day and a tabletop sound machine for sleep, although he was cautioned that different devices might be recommended once he saw the TRT provider. Distraction techniques were also recommended to help take his mind off his tinnitus. He used the hearing aids, sleep device and distraction techniques consistently. At his one month check-up, he reported significant improvement in his coping. He decided not to proceed with TRT.

Case 41: He developed slight tinnitus and distressing sound sensitivity after an accident. He loved music and socializing with friends. He found the sound from his usual activities bothered him, and at times, certain very loud noises around him would trigger a loud squealing tinnitus in his ears. He stopped playing piano and guitar, and stopped going out to restaurants or nightclubs. He began using earplugs and earmuffs all the time, and eventually became restricted to staying in his home where he could keep everything really quiet. He became frustrated and angry that his sound sensitivity prevented him from living a normal life and doing things he enjoyed.

Eventually he went to a tinnitus specialist who did a complete tinnitus evaluation. He received education and reassurance that there was treatment available. His care provider put together a treatment plan for him that included sound therapy and counselling therapy. The sound therapy included using pink noise and gradually re-introducing regular sound into his environment as well as gradually switching over to using appropriate hearing protection as needed. The counselling therapy included ongoing reassurance and specific techniques to help him stop reacting negatively to sound. He followed treatment recommendations, and over time the treatment was successful. Through treatment, he was able to return to the activities and lifestyle he enjoyed. His quality of life and ability to cope improved dramatically with the combination of sound therapy and counselling therapy (mind enrichment).

MIND ENRICHMENT

Men are disturbed not by things, but by views which they take of them. Epicetus.

JUST DON'T THINK ABOUT IT

The term tinnitus distress covers the variety of emotions experienced by any individual in response to their tinnitus. The mixture of emotions may include sadness, depression, anger, anxiety, fear, annoyance, irritability, guilt, etc. The scientific research clearly demonstrates that tinnitus distress is not related to tinnitus pitch or loudness, amount of hearing loss, or presence of sound sensitivity. The primary factor related to tinnitus distress is not the tinnitus sound itself, but the severity of the person's negative emotional reaction to their tinnitus sound.

Often people are told by well meaning folks (friends, families, health care providers) to "just stop thinking about it", "stop worrying" or "cheer up, it could be worse". One doctor told the author "if hearing loss were like having no feet, then tinnitus was like having no shoes". In other words, it might be uncomfortable, but it's not that bad. This advice did nothing to ease my negative reaction to the non-stop screeching with no end in sight. I continued to have constant negative thoughts about my tinnitus. I was not provided with any strategies to help me change my negative reaction and negative thoughts towards the tinnitus.

When therapy is needed, many people successfully use sound enrichment. However, people often continue to have negative reactions to their tinnitus even when using sound enrichment. Typically this is for two reasons. First, most people can still hear their tinnitus even when using sound enrichment. This is because sound is set at a soft to moderate comfortable loudness that often does not completely cover up the tinnitus. Second, for many people it is difficult to just stop reacting negatively to a chronic condition like tinnitus. Sound therapy or sound enrichment is a helpful treatment approach for coping better with the sounds of silence. Counselling therapy or mind enrichment is an effective treatment tool for coping better with the emotional side of tinnitus distress. This type of treatment can also help people distressed by sound sensitivity.

Sounds of Silence (Tinnitus) *is treated with* **Sound Enrichment**

Negative Emotional Reaction *is treated with* **Mind Enrichment**

Tinnitus is a chronic condition that is not expected to go away. People need tools to help them manage or cope over time. As discussed in previous chapters, tinnitus is often compared to chronic pain because they have a lot in common: they are invisible and long lasting. In fact, many people are dealing with both conditions. There is a higher incidence of chronic pain in people with tinnitus (e.g. headache, body pain, jaw pain). Pain and tinnitus also fluctuate up and down for no apparent rhyme or reason. They can vary from hour to hour or from day to day. This is a normal part of the nature of the beast. This can also lead to similar distress for tinnitus or chronic pain.

There are various techniques proven to work for people with chronic pain that are also proven to work for people with tinnitus. The goal of these techniques is to help reduce or eliminate any negative emotional reaction to the chronic condition. Treatment for tinnitus (or sound sensitivity) should not always focus on the ears. For many people, treatment needs to help reduce negative emotional reactions. But it is extremely difficult to directly change our emotions. As discussed in the chapter on How We Hear Tinnitus, our emotions or feelings are reflected in our background thoughts, inner voice or self-talk. So treatment needs to focus on the thoughts that underlie our emotions.

For example, it is snowing outside. One person thinks, "I can hardly wait to go for a walk in the snow". Their emotional reaction is positive. Another person thinks, "I'm scared to drive home. What if I get in an accident?" Their emotional reaction is negative. It is our thoughts that lead to whether we have a negative or positive emotional reaction. The same idea applies to having tinnitus. One person thinks, "Good thing I know about using sound enrichment." Their emotional reaction is positive. Another person thinks, "What if my tinnitus gets any louder? It will drive me nuts." Their emotional reaction is negative. Having tinnitus does not cause the emotion. The emotional reaction is a result of how the person thinks about the tinnitus. Often people may have developed a habit of thinking and reacting negatively towards their tinnitus.

Negative thoughts often include "what if" thinking. People with tinnitus distress often think about various "what if" scenarios that were described in the chapter on How We Hear Tinnitus. These include "What if I have a serious illness?" and "What if I can't live with it?" Most people are not trained to handle "what if" thinking that can lead to increased worry, anxiety, stress and difficulty coping.

When you think about your tinnitus, are your thoughts healing or hopeful? Or are you being overcome by "what if" thoughts or overcome at times where you can't stop thinking about or worrying over tinnitus? It is very possible to directly change these thoughts, especially with professional help. Just as a person can treat tinnitus sound with other sound, a person can also treat tinnitus thoughts with other thoughts.

FORMAL COUNSELLING THERAPY

At least some amount of counselling is recommended for people with any distress from tinnitus or sound sensitivity. People with mild distress often just need education and reassurance counselling by an audiologist after a tinnitus evaluation to ease any worry, concern or negative thoughts. People with moderate to severe distress may need additional counselling therapy from their audiologist or tinnitus specialist. Severely distressed people usually need more formal intensive counselling therapy. This may be obtained through a tinnitus specialist although people can also benefit from seeing a counselling specialist (e.g. psychologist, psychiatrist). Counselling specialists are far more widely available than tinnitus specialists. Counselling therapy usually takes a series of sessions (e.g. over a 2 to 3 month period).

Some people are reluctant to consider counselling therapy especially if referral to a psychologist or counselling specialist is recommended. But psychological techniques target emotional distress (e.g. anxiety, sadness, negative feelings, difficulty sleeping, etc.), and the techniques are just as helpful in managing tinnitus or sound sensitivity related emotional distress. Also many people with tinnitus have significant depression or sadness. Research shows that people who are depressed find their tinnitus to be more severe. Psychologists or counselling specialists can be a good resource to help.

Any counselling treatment is intended to help people cope better with life's difficulties so that they have an improved quality of life. Counselling therapy approaches used for tinnitus or sound sensitivity include but are certainly not limited to directive counselling, self regulation therapy, existential therapy, rational emotive behaviour therapy, and cognitive behaviour therapy. Therapists may specialize in one approach or select from various techniques or approaches depending on the individual person's needs. The focus of this chapter is a description of the most commonly used counselling approaches for tinnitus or sound sensitivity: directive counselling and cognitive behaviour therapy. This information is not meant to replace individual counselling therapy from a trained professional. It just gives some very basic information about some of the options available. Other approaches may also be used depending on your counselling specialist.

Directive Counselling is used in Tinnitus Retraining Therapy (TRT) in combination with sound therapy. Sound therapy was discussed in the chapter on Sound Enrichment. Directive counselling includes specific educational information to help get rid of any fear about tinnitus. A modified version sometimes called Auditory Retraining Therapy is used to treat sound sensitivity. The idea is for a person to stop having negative emotional reactions to tinnitus or sound. TRT is typically available from tinnitus specialists although sometimes other professionals (e.g. some counselling specialists) also have specific training in this method.

Cognitive Behaviour Therapy (CBT) or Cognitive Behavioural Therapy has been found successful for people with tinnitus. CBT could also help people dealing with sound sensitivity. This type of therapy helps people examine how their thoughts affect their emotions. Cognitive Behaviour Therapy is usually provided by psychologists or counselling specialists to help people cope better with chronic conditions, stress, fear, anxiety, and depression. This type of treatment is reported to reduce distress, and improve well-being and quality of life. Progressive Tinnitus Management (PTM) uses a CBT approach in combination with sound therapy. The four main Cognitive Behaviour Therapy techniques that can be used alone or in combination are cognitive, distraction, relaxation and imagination mind enrichment.

COGNITIVE MIND ENRICHMENT

We all have a stream of thoughts going on inside ourselves. For example, when you wake up you might think, "I don't want to get up yet". You might notice your tinnitus or sound sensitivity and think, "Today is going to be awful." This is sometimes called "self talk". Self-talk often represents negative thought patterns, particularly when people are dealing with chronic conditions such as tinnitus. Negative self-talk (including "what if" thinking) may reflect doubts and fears about our ability to cope. Cognitive mind enrichment or cognitive therapy is counselling therapy that helps people focus on their thoughts and change any negative thinking. It is used to help depression, anxiety, fear and other tinnitus related concerns. Therapy may be offered by counselling specialists in individual or group sessions.

The focus is not to change people into a "Pollyanna" type full of sunshiny positive thinking. The goal is to change from unhelpful negative thinking to helpful realistic neutral or positive thinking. Some experts explain this using a traffic light analogy. Red means the thought is unhelpful; it makes you feel upset and should be stopped. Green means the thought is helpful; it doesn't make you feel upset. "Today is going to be awful" is an unhelpful red thought. Over the course of treatment, a person's self-talk can change to a helpful green thought like "Good thing I have coping strategies I can use". This process is sometimes compared to weeding a garden. With the guidance of a counselling specialist, unhelpful negative thoughts are plucked out like weeds.

Sometimes people may also avoid certain activities because they have negative thoughts about what might happen. People often predict that they will have a problem (e.g. My tinnitus will be worse if I go out in my car, etc.). Some people with distressing tinnitus or sound sensitivity become isolated as they make excuses to avoid social and work activities that they fear will make things worse. In cognitive therapy, the counselling specialist helps encourage people to try activities. For example, a person may be worried about going out to see a movie at a movie theatre because they think it will be too loud. They could try seeing a movie that doesn't have a lot of loud special effects (e.g. gunfire, explosions) and see if the volume was still too loud. They could go see a movie but wear appropriate hearing protection and see if that would be comfortable enough at least every now and then. They could choose to watch a special movie at home set to a comfortable volume. The counselling specialist helps guide people through this process while problem solving any concerns that come up.

DISTRACTION MIND ENRICHMENT

There is an expression that what you focus on increases. It is certainly true that the more people focus on their tinnitus (or sound sensitivity), the more distressing it can become. Some authors describe a mental condition sometimes called "flow state". Flow state is the opposite of focusing. Flow state can be described as being on automatic pilot. For example, imagine you are driving home from the store. It is a trip you have taken many times. You reach your driveway, and realize you can't remember the drive. You were in flow state. Your body functioned automatically and your background thoughts were free to roam. In contrast, imagine you are driving home from the store in the middle of a fierce storm. All your thoughts are completely focused on each part of the trip. Each turn of the steering wheel. Each touch on the gas or brakes. You arrive home exhausted from the stress of worrying over the drive.

Tinnitus distress is strongly related to the amount of time people spend listening to their tinnitus and thinking about it. Some people with tinnitus rarely think about it, and for them it is not a problem. Other people find it difficult to focus on anything else because they are always thinking about their tinnitus. When you worry over tinnitus like a dog with a bone, then flow state is lost. When people regularly focus on their tinnitus, it leads to increased stress, anxiety and depression. It is essential to do all that you can to spend less time checking on and thinking about your tinnitus. However, this can be a hard habit to break. Distraction mind enrichment can help. While cognitive mind enrichment uses strategies to help a person think differently about their tinnitus, distraction mind enrichment uses strategies to help a person turn their thoughts away from their tinnitus.

One of the best ways not to think about tinnitus is to think about something else. This is because it is hard for people to focus on more than one thing at a time. Counselling specialists can teach people specific distraction techniques that can help them shift their focus away from their tinnitus. There are various distraction methods or techniques available. Counselling specialists usually help people try different methods so they can find the ones that work best for them. By using distraction mind enrichment techniques, the goal over time is to think less and less about the tinnitus until you reach the end of the day and realize you haven't had any particular thoughts about it. Outside of formal counselling therapy, there are distraction strategies that people can use in their daily life. These could include neutral thoughts, laughter, and informal distraction techniques.

J. L. Mayes

Neutral thoughts can be used to help focus attention and thoughts away from tinnitus. The idea is to get tinnitus off your mind. Many people come up with their own methods of distracting their thoughts to something specific. The following alphabet distraction and strange distraction are just a few ideas.

The alphabet distraction lets you distract your thoughts to a neutral topic. It can be used anytime you find it hard to stop thinking about your tinnitus. It is a technique the author learned at an Arthritis Society of Canada self-management program on coping with chronic pain that the author found also worked for her tinnitus. For the alphabet distraction, use every letter of the alphabet in order if possible. Choose any category you like such as girl's names, fruits or vegetables, flowers, countries, etc. Then work your way through the alphabet letter by letter. Don't worry if you can't think of something, just move on to the next letter. For example, if the category was animals, then a person might think of a = ant, b = bear, c = cat, d = dog, e = can't think of anything, f = frog, g = giraffe and so on. The key is that you are forcing yourself to think about something neutral instead of your tinnitus. With regular practice people often find that in the middle of doing the alphabet distraction, their thoughts automatically stray to other things (e.g. plans for the day, what they're going to cook for dinner, etc.). By regularly practicing thinking about something different, it becomes easier to stop your thoughts from settling on tinnitus.

Another distraction technique might be called the strange distraction. This is how it works. Sit down. Lift your right foot an inch above the ground. Start rotating it clockwise. Now use your right index finger to trace a figure eight in the air in front of you. Once you can do these actions simultaneously, you will likely have spent some time not thinking about your tinnitus.

Laughter can be good for a person's health and sense of well-being. Norman Cousins wrote a book called *Anatomy of an Illness as Perceived by the Patient,* which describes how he took charge of a disease through a combination of humour and treatment. It is hard to think about concerns or problems while you are laughing. Formal laughter therapy is done by certified "laughter leaders" who use the power of laughter to lift spirits, heal, and bring better physical health. Laughter and breathing exercises are often used. You can add laughter into your life by seeking out what makes you laugh. Choose funny television shows or comedy movies to watch. Find reading material that is funny. Some people even take a short "news break" and temporarily stop watching or reading the news to avoid reacting to the sad, negative or unpleasant things happening outside their community. It is okay to shift your focus to things that are light-hearted or humorous.

Making yourself smile and laugh even when you don't really feel happy are also effective techniques for battling anxiety, depression and stress. Grin at yourself in the mirror each morning as you get ready for the day. Practice making yourself laugh. Some experts call this fake it 'til you make it. As Zen master Thich Nhat Hanh once said, "Life is both dreadful and wonderful... Smiling means that we are ourselves, that we have sovereignty over ourselves, that we are not drowned in forgetfulness. How can I smile when I am filled with so much sorrow? It is natural—you need to smile to your sorrow because you are more than your sorrow." Whether you are genuinely happy or are just putting on a bit of a show to manage feeling down, smiles and laughter are an effective and inexpensive technique of distraction mind enrichment.

Informal Distraction Techniques can certainly help for tinnitus. The most commonly used informal distraction techniques involve keeping busy with enjoyable activities or hobbies. One of the worst things people can do is to stop participating in the activities that they enjoy. Sitting around doing nothing pleasant only leaves a person with a lot of time on their hands to think about their tinnitus. Call a friend or get going. The more you can keep yourself occupied with various activities or hobbies that you enjoy, the better you can be distracted. Try to identify when your tinnitus is more noticeable. During those times, keep busy with pleasant, meaningful activities, especially where you need to use your mind.

If you don't already have activities or hobbies that you participate in regularly, then find things to do that interest you and distract you from the tinnitus. For example, bird watching can be an interesting distraction, whether you have a birdfeeder in your garden or just look for different birds on a walk around your neighbourhood. Some people enjoy trying to identify the birds they see. But even just counting how many birds you see can be an easy neutral method of distracting your thoughts. Other examples might include exercise, cooking, reading, shopping, crafting, crossword puzzles, photography, gardening, fishing, golfing, woodworking, doing volunteer work. Activities or hobbies used will be as varied as the interests of different people with tinnitus.

RELAXATION MIND ENRICHMENT

Stress can make any chronic condition including tinnitus (or sound sensitivity) seem worse. It is sometimes unclear whether tinnitus makes people feel stressed and then distress increases, or whether stress makes tinnitus worse and then distress increases. As with the riddle of the chicken or the egg, it is not necessarily possible to tell whether the tinnitus or the stress came first. All that matters is that they often increase together. People can use relaxation mind enrichment techniques to help them feel less stressed, more relaxed, and better able to cope. Sometimes very distressed people have felt tense for so long that they have forgotten what it feels like to be relaxed or calm. Learning relaxation techniques can also help people know what it should feel like to be relaxed. Then they can better recognize when they are feeling tense, and when they need to use relaxation mind enrichment techniques.

Counselling specialists can teach people specific relaxation techniques that are often helpful in specific situations (e.g. sleep, stressful times, etc.). Usually people have a trial of different approaches under the guidance of their counselling specialist. This way they can try the techniques out and find the ones that work best for them. One commonly used technique is progressive muscle relaxation. With this technique, the counselling specialist teaches the person how to tense and relax all their different muscle groups in a specialized way to improve relaxation. Another body scan technique can be used to find tense muscle groups or areas in the body and then focus on relaxing that area.

Experts suggest that relaxation techniques are not as helpful if used on their own. They work best when used in combination with other mind enrichment techniques. Often counselling specialists incorporate distraction or imagination techniques into relaxation training. Some specialists will give their clients specially prepared relaxation tools (e.g. CD or DVD). Outside of formal treatment, relaxation strategies could include deep breathing, meditation, and informal relaxation techniques.

Deep Breathing has long been used as a method of improving relaxation. A counselling specialist can teach you proper deep breathing techniques. Deep breathing is also a component of certain types of stretching exercises. With deep breathing, you slowly breathe out as deeply as possible and then slowly breathe in as fully as possible. Usually deep breathing is done sitting or lying down in a comfortable position for a few minutes at a time (e.g. 5 to 10 minutes). Other people can't necessarily tell if you are using deep breathing.

So it is easy to practice during the day (e.g. while sitting at a stoplight in a car, during a television commercial, etc.). With practice, it is an effective relaxation technique to use before falling asleep or for when you are feeling stressed or tense.

Meditation has been used for centuries to reduce stress, anxiety and pain. Many cultures use meditation or contemplation to clear or empty the mind. Imagine the mind is like a pond full of water. If the water gets stirred up, it becomes cloudy. If the mind is constantly agitated, it also becomes cloudy or busy. If you take a glass of pond water and let it rest, the debris will sink to the bottom leaving the water clear. Similarly, if you take time to sit without agitating the mind, your thoughts will slow down and clear. When practiced regularly, meditation can calm the mind and bring feelings of relaxation and well-being.

Meditation is usually done in a quiet, peaceful place. However, people with tinnitus can benefit from using relaxation sound enrichment while they are meditating (e.g. water sounds, nature sounds, gentle instrumental music). There are many different types of meditation including deep breathing meditations. It is most helpful to start meditating with the support of a meditation teacher. People typically spend approximately 5 to 10 minutes on a meditation. Meditation works best when it is practiced regularly (e.g. daily or several times a week). If possible, choose a regular time of day to practice. Some people find that meditating at bedtime before falling asleep helps with relaxation.

Informal Relaxation Techniques can include various strategies or tools. Not everybody finds the same things relaxing, so specific techniques vary from person to person. The following examples are just a few ideas of what works for some people. Have a warm shower or bath. Go for a walk, or do some gentle exercises that make you feel good when you are finished. Hug somebody. Pet a dog or a cat. Have a nice cup of tea or a cool drink. Take 5 or 10 minutes and just sit or lie down in a pleasant place with no interruptions. Some people find using a swing relaxing (e.g. sitting on a garden swing or using a swing at a playground). Think about what makes you feel relaxed or at ease, and try to make a point of setting aside time to relax during your daily life.

There are also various tools available for home practice and use. These include books and audio or audio-visual devices like CDs or DVDs. They are usually under the categories of chronic pain, tinnitus or relaxation in libraries, book stores or stores. Tools may describe different relaxation techniques and walk a person through them step by step (e.g. progressive muscle relaxation, body scan, deep breathing, meditation, etc.).

IMAGINATION MIND ENRICHMENT

The formal term for imagination mind enrichment is guided imagery or visualization. It is a therapy technique used for various conditions including chronic pain. Imagination mind enrichment or guided imagery can help a person shift their attention to specific mental images or pictures instead of their tinnitus. Sometimes this is referred to as creating a calm inner oasis. It is important to practice regularly for this technique to be most effective. Some people will find guided imagery easier to do than other people. Counselling specialists can help a person become skilled at developing imaginative mental images or scenes that involve all the senses (e.g. sight, touch, hearing, smell, taste). People can learn to use pleasant imagery and/or tinnitus imagery.

For pleasant imagery, people imagine a scene that is enjoyable for them. For example, a person could imagine petting their cat. They could imagine how the cat looks, the softness of the fur, the sound of purring, the warm smell of the fur. With practice, people can use their imagination to picture various scenes to help take their mind off their tinnitus. Some people also use their imagination to picture pleasant memories. For example, people can remember a special vacation, an enjoyable family gathering, or favourite place in detail. Other people use their imagination by choosing a pleasant daydream. For example, what would your dream vacation be like, or how would you play each hole of your favourite golf course?

For tinnitus imagery, the idea is to imagine a scene that involves all the senses including sound effects similar to your tinnitus. For example, if your tinnitus sounds like a buzz, you might imagine bumblebees in a garden full of flowers. Counselling specialists can help you create a mental image that works best for your tinnitus sound. Another technique is to imagine tinnitus as something specific and then change it in some way. As you change your tinnitus image, the tinnitus may change. Your counselling specialist can help you think of an image to use for your tinnitus. Different people might think of images like an ear on fire, an angry hornet or a chainsaw. One person might imagine pouring water on the ear to put out the fire. Another person might imagine the angry hornet changing into a hummingbird. Or imagine squashing the hornet with a rolled up magazine. And another person might imagine the chainsaw turning into a soft power drill. Or imagine smashing the chainsaw to pieces with a sledgehammer.

Experts suggest that imagination techniques are not as helpful if used on their own. They work best when used in combination with other mind enrichment techniques. Outside of formal treatment, imagination strategies mainly include informal imagination techniques.

Informal Imagination Techniques include various tools available for home practice and use. These include books and audio or audio-visual devices like CDs or DVDs. They are usually under the categories of relaxation, meditation, or possibly creative visualization in libraries, book stores or stores. Tools may describe different image or visualization techniques and walk a person through them step by step. Sometimes people also use favourite pictures, paintings, or photographs of people or places that they love to help them create positive mental images to focus on.

Table 9
MIND ENRICHMENT OPTIONS

Cognitive Techniques (to control thought content)	• Directive counselling (Tinnitus Retraining Therapy) • Formal counselling therapy
Distraction Techniques (to change thought focus)	• Formal counselling therapy • Neutral thoughts • Laughter • Informal distraction techniques
Relaxation Techniques (to relax)	• Formal counselling therapy • Deep breathing • Meditation • Informal relaxation techniques
Imagination Techniques (to calm)	• Formal counselling therapy • Pleasant or tinnitus imagery • Informal imagination techniques

MIND ENRICHMENT PLAN

Counselling therapy or mind enrichment does not get rid of the tinnitus sound. This type of treatment just helps you change how you react to the sound. There is no single mind enrichment technique that will work best for everyone. Techniques are usually most successful when planned and used with the guidance of a professional counselling specialist or tinnitus specialist. If you are in formal therapy, then your care provider will give you counselling and specific treatment approaches for your tinnitus or sound sensitivity.

It is important to remember that mind enrichment techniques are coping skills that need to be practiced and used in daily life to be most helpful. Usually people practice techniques approximately 10 minutes a day (or as recommended by their care provider) to improve their ability to use the technique effectively. Often cognitive techniques work best when people are having negative thoughts. Distraction techniques work best when tinnitus is grabbing people's attention. Relaxation techniques work best when people are feeling tense or anxious. And imagination techniques work best to relax or calm the mind. It is helpful to practice the four main techniques (cognitive, distraction, relaxation, imagination) so people know what works best for them in different situations. For example, during the day, a person might use cognitive or distraction techniques, and then use relaxation or imagination techniques before falling asleep.

Mind enrichment techniques help lead to a decrease in the amount of time spent focusing on tinnitus or sound sensitivity. By changing our thoughts, it is possible to reduce or eliminate any negative emotional reaction. This can help people feel more in control. It may also help the emotional center of the brain reset itself by becoming less active or less responsive. This in turn can lower anxiety, fear, and stress. The result is a sense of greater well-being and improved quality of life.

Mind enrichment may be used alone although it is most commonly used in combination with sound enrichment for a more effective comprehensive treatment. Sound enrichment (treating sound with sound) and Mind enrichment (treating thoughts with thoughts) are helpful strategies to cope better. Sound enrichment allows you to keep your ears busy with replacement sounds so that tinnitus is changed, reduced or eliminated. Mind enrichment allows you to keep your mind busy with replacement thoughts, so that over time the habit of thinking about tinnitus is changed, reduced or eliminated.

Sound Enrichment

plus **Mind Enrichment**

equals **LESS TINNITUS DISTRESS**

A person might get both sound therapy and counselling therapy from a tinnitus specialist. In other cases a person's audiologist can do education and reassurance counselling, and then if necessary can refer them to a counselling specialist for a well-rounded treatment approach. The audiologist can then focus on sound enrichment including fitting of any hearing aids or devices, while the counselling specialist can focus on mind enrichment techniques.

There is no doubt that counselling therapy helps people with tinnitus or sound sensitivity. If you are in counselling therapy, you must be motivated since formal counselling treatment takes persistence and hard work. As with other treatment methods, counselling therapy or mind enrichment requires guidance, practice and time before you'll begin to notice any benefit. But mind enrichment is worth it when the end result is reduced distress and better coping.

Author's Case: I have normal hearing and had severe tinnitus distress. I have never attended formal counselling therapy for my tinnitus. I used to think about my tinnitus all the time constantly checking to see how it was doing, what the loudness was like compared to the day before, how the loudness was changing during the day, etc. Barely a minute went by that I wasn't listening to and thinking about my tinnitus whether I was working, reading, watching TV, etc. My thoughts were very negative (e.g. I wish this would go away, If this gets any louder, I won't be able to take it any more, etc.). As I learned more about mind enrichment or counselling therapy approaches, I realized that my habit of constantly listening to and thinking about my tinnitus was completely counter productive. If anything, it was making my tinnitus worse.

I had used distraction techniques to deal with pain, and decided to use similar techniques for my tinnitus. I began using the alphabet distraction every time I found myself listening to or thinking about my tinnitus. I can name fruits and vegetables from A to Z. I can also do girls names, boys names, capital cities, countries, flowers, and various other categories. It is one of the hardest things I have ever done, but

I forced my thoughts away from my tinnitus. During this time I also began using sound enrichment, so it helped that the extra sound in my environment made my tinnitus less noticeable and attention grabbing. I also tried to fill my days with activities that I enjoyed (e.g. walks, swimming, biking, gardening, watching my birdfeeder, playing piano, golfing, etc.).

After a period of months, I noticed that my thoughts began shifting automatically to various topics depending on my upcoming plans and activities. My thoughts no longer went immediately and constantly to my tinnitus. I gradually stopped needing to use the specific alphabet distraction technique. My tinnitus was still there, but the majority of the time I didn't even stop to think about it. The exception was in the morning waking up and at night falling asleep. When I listened to my tinnitus at those times, I kept it to a minimum (a few seconds) and just acknowledged it with a neutral thought (e.g. I hear you, or Yup, still there). Perhaps I should consider some additional counselling therapy, since for some reason I do think of my tinnitus as a "you" instead of an "it". Probably since we've been hanging out together for so long.

Since my personality has a tendency towards worry, anxiety and depression (regardless of my tinnitus), I also use relaxation techniques when I feel stressed. Deep breathing is very helpful for me. I also find progressive muscle relaxation helpful especially before falling asleep. It is relaxing and helps calm my thoughts. I also take "news breaks" regularly. During these times I don't watch TV news since it is often negative or unhappy. I don't need to know about every horrible thing that happens in the world. I stay informed about major world and local events through the radio and my community newspaper. I find this gives me good sources of information that includes lighthearted and funny stories that often go unreported in the mainstream media.

Mind enrichment is definitely an effective treatment tool to consider. Through a combination of mind enrichment and sound enrichment techniques, my tinnitus does not distress me very often.

Case 42: He had moderate to severe tinnitus. He considered Tinnitus Retraining Therapy and Cognitive Behavioural Therapy as treatment options. He would have had a long travel distance to attend TRT, so he chose a counselling specialist in his local area that offered CBT. The therapist worked with him on cognitive and distraction therapy techniques. They also worked with him on relaxation techniques and gave him a specific relaxation CD that he could use at home. They worked on some guided imagery techniques, although he did not find those as helpful. Overall, he found the CBT gave him control over his tinnitus, and helped to greatly improve his coping ability. He returned for follow-ups as needed when he had difficulty coping with tinnitus flare-ups due to life events (e.g. death in the family).

Case 43: She had tinnitus, and was worried it meant she was losing her hearing. After a tinnitus evaluation, her audiologist explained how tinnitus was a benign, natural and common symptom. She learned that she had hearing loss that was causing her hearing difficulties. She decided to have a trial period with hearing aids. She did not need any additional counselling beyond basic education and reassurance.

Case 44: He had severe tinnitus after suffering a head injury. His audiologist gave him education and reassurance about tinnitus. He was not interested in any formal counselling therapy or specific distraction, relaxation or imagination techniques. He began regularly volunteering at a support group for people with head injuries. He reported that this helped take his mind off his tinnitus. He also used sound enrichment.

Case 45: She had hearing loss and sound sensitivity. She attended Tinnitus Retraining Therapy. She received directive counselling and specific sound therapy. She noticed significant improvement over the course of therapy.

Case 46: He had tinnitus and hearing loss. He went to a tinnitus specialist for tinnitus music therapy (Neuromonics Tinnitus Treatment). As part of the treatment program, he also received education and counselling to help him cope better.

Case 47: He had normal hearing and tinnitus. He attended counselling for his tinnitus and learned various relaxation techniques that helped with sleep. He was frustrated because he loved hiking with his family, but he really noticed his tinnitus while hiking because it was so quiet outdoors. He found he was always thinking negative thoughts when hiking (e.g. What if my tinnitus bothers me so much I can't hike with my family any more?) The relaxation techniques he had learned didn't help. Sound enrichment was considered, but he wanted to hear the sounds around him (e.g. nature, conversation), and didn't want to add in extra sound or music through a wearable personal listening system.

The tinnitus specialist recommended distraction techniques to help re-focus his thoughts (e.g. try pleasant conversation with hiking companions; try identifying birds or animals from their sounds or tracks; try counting or identifying plants, birds, or animals along the hike; try rock hunting along the trail if interested; try the walking distraction or the alphabet distraction (e.g. A to Z wish list of places to hike).

Other specific distraction techniques were also discussed. For example, while hiking try to imagine describing the hike to someone. What landmarks could he tell them about? What specific colours and shades would describe things around him (e.g. the ground, plants, sky, people, animals, etc.)? What sensations is he feeling (e.g. crunch of trail underfoot, warmth of sun on skin)? What can he smell along the hike (e.g. crushed foliage, dirt, etc.)? What is his favourite part of the hike? The idea would be to focus thoughts and images on the enjoyable hike itself. This could even be used later to remember as pleasant imagery visualization.

Case 48: She had hearing loss and distressing tinnitus. Her audiologist helped her with a Progressive Tinnitus Management style sound enrichment plan including hearing aids for day and audiobooks for night set loud enough to hear the voice reading but not necessarily make out the words. She began doing gentle exercising while listening to enjoyable music. Her audiologist referred her to a psychologist experienced in CBT to help her with anxiety, depression and insomnia she was having because of her tinnitus. She noticed significant improvement in her coping abilities and sense of well-being.

Case 49: He had severe tinnitus that sounded like a train whistle. He went to a counselling specialist. He found one effective tool for him was using tinnitus imagery. He would imagine a mountain scene with a railroad track running through it with a train whistling away. He found with practice this helped change his thoughts about his tinnitus to be more neutral. He used this technique at least once a day as directed by his counselling specialist. He also learned to use helpful distraction techniques. For sleep or other times when he was feeling stressed or anxious, he used relaxation techniques including deep breathing. He also began using body enrichment techniques.

BODY ENRICHMENT

Seize fate by the throat. Ludwig van Beethoven.

Maximizing health can maximize ability to cope with tinnitus. Body enrichment means improving your health as much as possible. As discussed in the chapter on Treatment Planning, tinnitus is associated with various ear, medical and dental conditions. It is important to work with the appropriate health care professional to treat any existing conditions. Since there is a higher incidence of pain (e.g. headache, neck pain, back or shoulder pain, jaw pain, etc.) in people with tinnitus, treatment for pain may also be a consideration. The overall tinnitus treatment team may include doctors, ear specialists, dentists, physiotherapists, chiropractors and/or massage therapists.

In many cases there is no specific medical treatment for people with tinnitus. Appropriate exercise, diet and a healthy lifestyle can all maximize health, improve coping ability, and reduce tinnitus distress. The focus of this chapter is body enrichment ideas that may be helpful for anyone with tinnitus. People with sound sensitivity could also benefit from body enrichment.

EXERCISE

Many tinnitus experts recommend keeping your body busy to help cope better with tinnitus. In addition to the physical benefits, exercise can distract your attention from your tinnitus, reduce stress and anxiety, improve mood, and help with relaxation. It is important to get clearance from your doctor before starting any exercise program. Exercise does not have to mean major athletics or aerobics. Gentle activities such as walking, swimming or yoga are effective.

Many people with tinnitus find these forms of exercise are helpful not only for flexibility, strength and cardiovascular fitness, but also for improving their sense of overall well-being. Laughter is also good exercise. Some experts suggest that one minute of laughing gets your heart rate up as much as 10 minutes on a rowing machine. Sometimes people notice their tinnitus temporarily increases after exercise, especially after a cardiovascular workout when their heart rate has been safely elevated. The benefit of exercise usually outweighs any temporary change. Check with your doctor if you have any concerns.

DIET

There are various foods and drinks that have been shown to worsen tinnitus in some people. For that reason, people with tinnitus are sometimes advised to avoid certain food (e.g. sugar, salt, chocolate) and drinks including beverages with alcohol or caffeine (e.g. coffee, tea, cola). But something that affects one person's tinnitus may have absolutely no effect on somebody else. Many people won't change their diet if the change will increase distress at the loss of something nice (e.g. enjoying a chocolate bar, cup of coffee or glass of wine).

Some people change their diet by cutting out certain food or drinks to see if their tinnitus improves. After approximately a week, people then try the food or drink again to see if it affects their tinnitus. The potential problem is that tinnitus fluctuates so much for no particular reason that it is hard to tell if any improvement is from the diet change or just a normal tinnitus change. People usually need to repeat the process a couple of times to see if the food or drink is really affecting the tinnitus. If it turns out that a food or drink does affect the tinnitus, people can make the decision whether they want to change their diet all or some of the time.

Caffeine commonly increases tinnitus for many people. It is found in coffee, tea, and chocolate, but may also be in unexpected products such as energy drinks and some types of mints. If you are sensitive to caffeine, make sure you read labels carefully. If you need to reduce or eliminate your caffeine intake, do it gradually to help avoid "withdrawal headaches". In other words, don't go overnight from 12 cups of coffee daily to zero cups of coffee. Instead, you may wish to eliminate a cup of coffee a day over a period of weeks until your caffeine intake is reduced to a reasonable amount (e.g. one to three cups a day) or no caffeine at all if you are very sensitive. If you are able to enjoy reasonable amounts of caffeine, don't drink or consume it within 6 hours of bedtime otherwise sleep may be affected.

J. L. Mayes

Some research suggests that certain people with tinnitus may be low in B Vitamins, magnesium or zinc. Taking these vitamins and minerals helps a limited number of people with tinnitus. Try to find natural food sources or consider taking a regular daily vitamin and mineral supplement to maintain healthy levels of B vitamins, magnesium and zinc in your system. It is not recommended that people with tinnitus take "mega-doses" of any supplement. Your doctor or pharmacist can guide you in selecting a multi-vitamin and mineral supplement appropriate for you.

It is also suggested that certain herbal supplements (e.g. Gingko Biloba, St. John's Wort) may help some people with tinnitus. There is currently no conclusive scientific research to support claims that these herbs are effective for tinnitus, although some individuals find them helpful. Caution should be taken when taking any herbal supplements since they can have side effects (e.g. cardiovascular related) and may interact badly with prescription drugs. Anyone considering taking an herbal supplement should get clearance from his or her doctor first. Make sure any doctors or care providers you see for any reason are aware of everything you are taking including herbal remedies. Herbal supplements may not be permitted in combination with some formal tinnitus treatment programs.

HEALTHY LIFESTYLE

People's lifestyle can certainly affect their ability to cope with their tinnitus or sound sensitivity. There are huge amounts of information currently available on diet and lifestyle choices that are considered healthy. Avoid fads and trends. Eat healthy. Drink lots of water. Don't smoke. Anything in excess (e.g. caffeine, alcohol) has the potential to affect health and increase distress. Moderation is the key. Make lifestyle choices that make you feel good.

> **Author's Case:** I have normal hearing and had severe tinnitus distress. Sound enrichment and mind enrichment have made the most difference to my tinnitus perception and ability to cope. I try to eat healthy, and take daily multi-vitamin and mineral supplements that include B Vitamins, magnesium and zinc. I have tried taking Gingko Biloba in the past. After several weeks of taking it daily as recommended on the package, I noticed a slight decrease in the loudness of my tinnitus. When the package was finished, I did not continue with it. The small benefit I noticed was not enough for me to keep taking this herbal

supplement on a regular basis, although it could be useful during flare-ups. I exercise regularly including walking, biking, yoga, and swimming. I have also taken Flamenco dancing. This is a surprisingly noisy activity between the music, clapping, stamping and castanets (which sound like crazed woodpeckers in the hands of amateurs). Although my tinnitus was temporarily louder after dance lessons, the exercise and enjoyment was worth it for me. I feel better and sleep better when I exercise. I believe Body Enrichment helps improve my overall coping ability from day to day.

Case 50: He had moderate tinnitus. Every evening he and his wife prepared a gourmet meal at home, and enjoyed it with a glass of wine. He would feel angry and resentful towards his tinnitus if he stopped drinking wine because of it. He found the daily special meal helped him feel good and cope better.

Case 51: She used hearing aids for a severe to profound hearing loss and had mild to moderate tinnitus that she was coping well with. She began noticing her tinnitus increasing in loudness until it became almost unbearable. She and her audiologist worked together to try to figure out a solution. The only thing she could think of was that a few months previously she had started to take one baby aspirin daily for heart disease prevention. After getting approval from her doctor, she tried cutting out the aspirin for a week and then re-introducing it. She did this several times. Each time she stopped taking aspirin, she noticed her tinnitus loudness decreased. She stopped taking aspirin completely for several months, and her tinnitus settled down. The low dose aspirin was a tinnitus aggravator for her.

Case 52: She had received tinnitus music therapy for her severe tinnitus, and was coping well. Then she had a severe flare up. After consulting with her tinnitus specialist, she realized that the flare-up happened after she had eaten large amounts of chocolate over a period of weeks. When she stopped eating chocolate, her tinnitus settled back down. If she ate chocolate, she could expect her tinnitus to be aggravated. She decided to just eat it on special occasions, and live with the flare-up.

Case 53: He began to have distressing tinnitus. A tinnitus evaluation identified moderate tinnitus and a high frequency hearing loss. He was referred for a medical evaluation before any tinnitus treatment was considered. His family doctor diagnosed him with diabetes. Once his diabetes was under control, his tinnitus settled down. No specific tinnitus treatment was needed. He ended up getting hearing aids for his hearing loss.

Case 54: She was in Tinnitus Retraining Therapy for her severe tinnitus. She heard that St. John's Wort could be helpful, and began taking it. When she discussed this with her TRT provider, they recommended that she stop taking any herbal supplement since it was not appropriate in combination with TRT. She decided to continue with TRT, and stopped taking the herb. Over time, she noticed improvement in her tinnitus coping with the TRT program.

Case 55: He had moderate tinnitus and hearing loss. He used sound enrichment and mind enrichment techniques. He also decided to try joining a swim club since he had always enjoyed swimming. He really enjoyed the practices, swim meets, and social events. He looked forward to the swim club activities, and found they helped take his mind off his tinnitus. He also found the exercise tired him out, so his sleep really improved as well.

Case 56: He had severe tinnitus. He tried to make sure he carried on with all the activities that he enjoyed. He began biking regularly and drinking more water each day. He noticed his tinnitus much less over time.

Case 57: He had moderate tinnitus. He worked in a job where he was on his feet all day. After work he just wanted to do nothing, but that was when he really noticed his tinnitus. By bedtime, he found it hard to fall asleep. His wife wanted him to go for walks with her in the evening, but he felt he got enough exercise at work. His audiologist talked to him about the benefits of walking for tinnitus and improved sleep. They also discussed the benefits of pleasant company and conversation during an evening walk that could help distract him from his tinnitus. He decided to start going for walks with his wife after work. He found he began noticing his tinnitus less in the evening. He also started to use sound enrichment in the evenings as well as using sleep management techniques.

SLEEP MANAGEMENT

To sleep, perchance to dream. William Shakespeare (Hamlet).

There are various things that can disturb anybody's sleep including aging, pain, or sleep disorders. However, tinnitus can also disturb sleep for many people. When anything interferes with the usual patterns or cycles of sleep, a person can feel tired or not rested. Over 50% of people report problems sleeping because of their tinnitus. Often people with the greatest distress have tinnitus and sleep problems. Sleep difficulties can include difficulty falling asleep, waking up in the middle of the night and finding it hard to get back to sleep, waking too early or feeling tired when waking up in the morning, early morning headaches and depression. These difficulties can cause increased stress and anxiety that make it harder to cope with tinnitus.

It is important to remember that sleep difficulties are very common even in people who don't have tinnitus. There are various strategies that can help anyone (with or without tinnitus) sleep better. These general guidelines are described in various books and Websites on improving sleep. Ideas include:

- Get up at the same time every morning. This is the most important rule for promoting good sleep. It is the best way to set your internal "clock" and regulate sleeping and waking times.

- Avoid naps. Napping disrupts your internal "clock" and decreases the quality and quantity of sleep at night.

- Keep the alarm clock turned away from you. Clock-watching promotes wakefulness rather than sleepiness.

- Go to bed only when you feel sleepy.

- Take a warm bath (not hot) before going to bed.

- Give yourself 20 minutes to fall asleep. If you have not fallen asleep then get up and do something relaxing or slightly monotonous.

- Have a cool, dark, comfortable bedroom.

- Keep regular rituals and routines before bedtime. This helps to reinforce sleepiness. For example, read one chapter of a book every night while lying in bed.

- Avoid caffeine, alcohol and tobacco in the evening (e.g. for at least 6 hours before bedtime).

- Exercise moderately in the late afternoon or early evening.

- Unwind long before bedtime. Leave your worries at the bedroom door.

- Save your bedroom for pleasure, relaxation and sleep. Work projects, studying, budgeting, eating, arguing, etc. are best done elsewhere.

In addition to these sleep strategies, there are also tinnitus specific strategies to improve sleep. Strategies include sound enrichment, mind enrichment, body enrichment, prescription drugs, and sleep disorder treatment.

SOUND ENRICHMENT

Experts on tinnitus recommend sound enrichment to help improve sleep for people with tinnitus who have sleep difficulties. Many people with tinnitus have sleep problems that leave them exhausted, stressed, and anxious. They have difficulty coping with their family, social and work commitments because they are tired. In general, people with distressing tinnitus and sleep problems fall into two main groups. There is one group of people who "will do anything". These people are open to using sound enrichment to help them sleep and cope better. Then there is the second group. These people say they have difficulties sleeping because of their tinnitus. But when sound enrichment for sleep is recommended, their response is "but I like it quiet".

Many people think that quiet or silence is the best option in dealing with their tinnitus. This is false, especially for sleep. Silence or quiet can be a poor sleep trap for people with tinnitus. If you want to trap a monkey, put a lid on a jar and poke a hole in the lid large enough for the monkey's hand. Put a banana in the jar. The monkey will reach in to get the banana, but the hole will be too big for the banana and the hand together. The monkey will refuse to release the banana. The monkey refuses to change its expectation, because it thinks if it keeps holding on that it will get the banana. The monkey stays stuck in the trap.

When people hold on to silence, they stay stuck in the trap of poor sleep. They incorrectly expect that if they keep holding on to silence, they might sleep better. People with tinnitus need to release the expectation of silence to escape the trap of sleep problems. As discussed in the chapter on Sound Enrichment, if you have sleep difficulties you need to use sound to treat tinnitus even when sleeping. Sleep sound helps you sleep soundly.

See chapter on Sound Enrichment for further details on sleep sound enrichment including sound types and sound machines that can be used to help with sleep. Some people select devices with battery back up so the device keeps working even if the power goes off. An audiologist or tinnitus specialist can help guide you in selecting the most appropriate sleep sound enrichment for your individual needs. Use sound set so that you can hear it in the background, but it is not loud enough to keep you awake. If you start to use sound enrichment for sleep and it seems to make your tinnitus worse, then set the loudness to a softer level. The level can always be gradually increased over time. Some sound is better than no sound. When using sound enrichment for sleep:

- Use a steady, neutral and monotonous sound type that you find relaxing or soothing.

- Try tabletop sound machines, bedside sound devices, air purifiers, fans, or other devices as recommended by your care provider.

- If necessary, plug your sound device into a pillow speaker to listen through.

- Turn the sound to a comfortable loudness level.

- Set the relaxation sound to run constantly throughout the night until you wake up. Never use a timer to shut off your relaxation sound enrichment during the night.

- Consider using distraction sound to fall asleep with a timer to turn it off after a certain period of time (e.g. TV or radio with automatic shut off) along with relaxation sound running continuously through the night.

- Use sound enrichment regularly every night.

Never use hearing protection for sleep. This creates sound reduction, which is the opposite of sound enrichment. Tinnitus often seems louder while wearing hearing protection, which is not helpful when trying to sleep. Over time, using hearing protection for sleep on a regular daily basis can also make tinnitus (and sound sensitivity) worse. See chapter on Hearing Protection Management for more information.

MIND ENRICHMENT

See chapter on Mind Enrichment for techniques that can be helpful for sleep. Distraction or imagination strategies help some people with falling asleep. Relaxation strategies are most commonly helpful. One interesting technique focuses on how we breathe. Ancient yoga masters (yogis) discovered how people naturally do not breathe evenly through their nostrils. We always breathe slightly more through one nostril than the other, and this changes constantly over the course of our day. Stronger right nostril breathing is associated with a logical or alert state of mind, and stronger left nostril breathing is associated with relaxation or a drowsy state of mind.

If a person is feeling anxious or stressed, they can gently press down and close off their right nostril so they are breathing mainly through the left nostril. This is reported to reduce anxiety or negative emotions. It could be a helpful technique to use at bedtime since it also increases drowsiness. When people lie down on their right side, this automatically shifts breathing more towards the left nostril. Since this promotes a relaxed state of mind, many people find that they fall asleep more deeply and quickly if they can go to sleep while lying on their right side. Of course we are all unique, and there are a few people who find the opposite right nostril breathing more relaxing. Other relaxation techniques described in the Mind Enrichment chapter are also known to help people fall asleep more easily and sleep better.

BODY ENRICHMENT

As discussed in the chapter on Body Enrichment, people with tinnitus can change their exercise, diet and lifestyle choices to improve their health with the additional benefit of improving sleep.

PRESCRIPTION DRUGS

Research suggests that the majority of people with sleep problems never discuss them with their doctor. This is unfortunate since medical treatment such as prescription drugs may be helpful. Some people try over the counter sleep aids or alternative remedies (e.g. Melatonin, Tryptophan, Valerian) that can still have side effects or interact with other medical treatment. Discuss any sleep problems and options available with your doctor. Prescription drugs may need to be considered. Keep in mind that some prescription drugs used for sleep can be addictive (e.g. benzodiazepam family) and in rare cases some may have the side effects of causing tinnitus or making tinnitus worse. Work closely with your doctor to find the best choice for you. Generally it takes months of using a sleep drug to notice the full effect on your system. Sleep drugs can help improve coping as people build up their individual treatment plan (e.g. sound enrichment, mind enrichment, body enrichment, etc.). Use of prescription drugs should only be phased out gradually under medical guidance. Keep track of which medications are helpful in case of future flare-ups (episodes of disturbed sleep).

SLEEP DISORDER TREATMENT

In some cases, people actually have trouble sleeping because of a sleep disorder rather than their tinnitus. If necessary, your doctor can refer you to a sleep specialist or sleep clinic for evaluation and treatment. Keep in mind that the person with tinnitus may have the sleep disorder. However, a partner with a sleep disorder may also disturb your sleep. The most common sleep disorders that can disturb sleep or make people feel tired after sleeping include snoring and sleep apnea. When the airways become partly blocked while sleeping, this can lead to the noise we call snoring. Sleep apnea is when a person stops breathing briefly but repeatedly while sleeping.

Over the counter "stop snoring" aids are available (e.g. strips that go on the nose). Air purifiers may improve bedroom air quality to help breathing, reduce mild snoring, and result in a more restful sleep. Formal medical treatment for snoring or sleep apnea includes surgery, airway machines, or dental appliances. The surgery is very painful and has a limited success rate. Airway machines that force air into the nose can be worn at night while a person is sleeping. Over half of people are able to keep using this type of machine regularly. Dental appliances are similar to appliances used to stop teeth grinding while sleeping. They are worn in the mouth while sleeping to hold the jaw in a position that helps keep airways as open as possible. These appliances are quite effective in stopping snoring and can help mild to moderate sleep apnea. A sleep specialist or sleep clinic can evaluate whether you have a sleep disorder and what treatment is appropriate for your individual situation.

SLEEP MANAGEMENT PLAN

Sleep management techniques can definitely help improve sleep. A combination of medical and non-medical treatment approaches may be most useful depending on the severity of the sleep problems. To summarize:

- Follow general guidelines for better sleep.

- Use constant comfortable relaxation sound enrichment in the bedroom. Distraction sound enrichment that shuts off automatically after falling asleep may also help some people.

- Use relaxation mind enrichment to reduce stress and promote relaxation. Distraction or imagination mind enrichment techniques may also help.

- Use body enrichment techniques to help your body prepare for sleep (e.g. exercise, avoid caffeine, etc.).

- If necessary on a temporary basis, use a non-addictive over the counter sleep medication or talk to your doctor about prescription drugs to help with sleep.

- If sleep problems continue, you (and your sleep partner if you have one) should go to a sleep clinic to evaluate and treat any sleep disorder.

Author's Case: I like it quiet. Despite knowing and seeing the benefits of sound enrichment for sleep, I didn't want to add sound into my bedroom. I was always very fatigued despite taking daily naps. Even though I felt so tired, I often lay in bed at night for hours trying to fall asleep, or would wake up in the middle of the night and take hours to get back to sleep. I found a good book on sleep at the public library, and began to follow guidelines. I bought room darkening drapes so that my bedroom was very dark at night. I stopped clock watching. I stopped napping. This was very difficult since I was exhausted and longed to nap. But over time I began to sleep better. On afternoons when I just couldn't stay awake and ended up taking a nap, I realized it took much longer to fall asleep and I didn't sleep as well. Now when I just have to have a nap, I limit it to an hour.

I also stopped drinking caffeine after 6:00 p.m. I try to exercise daily (e.g. walk), and sleep better when I do. I use a dental appliance at night to help with teeth grinding. Using the dental appliance reduces jaw pain for me, and I think it also helps reduce my tinnitus. I accept that every now and then I get insomnia for no particular reason. When I can't fall asleep or wake up in the middle of the night, I find deep breathing or progressive muscle relaxation helps make me feel more relaxed and sleepy. I have also started pressing down on my right nostril so I am only breathing through my left nostril for a few minutes after I lay down on my right side to sleep. I seem to fall asleep faster when I do this.

For many years, I was very resistant to using sleep sound enrichment. I have no good explanation for this other than stubbornness. Because of problems with allergies and asthma, my doctor ordered me to use an air purifier in my bedroom. The sound of the air purifier was very similar to white noise. It could be set to low for a soft sound or to high for a moderate sound. I began with the setting on low but after a few weeks starting turning it on high. I could still hear my tinnitus over the sound of the air purifier but the extra sound definitely made my tinnitus less noticeable than when my bedroom was completely quiet. The first benefit I noticed immediately was better sleep. I was breathing better because of the improved air quality, and more importantly the sound helped cover up my husband's snoring and sleep sounds. The gentle white type noise did not bother my husband at all. It may have covered up any of my sleep sounds for him too (although of course I don't snore).

After a period of several months, I realized that I could no longer hear my tinnitus over the sound of the air purifier. My tinnitus had significantly dropped in loudness. Using sleep sound enrichment has made the most dramatic improvement in my tinnitus coping and perception than any other technique I have used. My only regret is that I didn't start using it sooner. I will never stop using sound enrichment for sleep. When I am on vacation, I use fans or air conditioners if available in the room I am sleeping in. If no sound generating devices are available, then I don't use anything. I don't stress out over taking a short break. But hearing my tinnitus "full strength" without any sound enrichment at night makes me appreciate the benefit of sleep sound enrichment. I also notice that my tinnitus starts increasing in loudness the longer I stop using sound enrichment at night.

In addition to the "white noise" relaxation sound enrichment, I also watch TV at bedtime. I set the TV on a sleep timer so it shuts off automatically (doesn't run all night). Usually I fall asleep before the TV shuts off. This additional distraction sound is helpful for me when falling asleep. My only regret is that I didn't start using sound enrichment for sleep sooner. I believe it has made a profound difference in my tinnitus perception (reduced loudness) and my ability to cope.

Case 58: He had tinnitus, but did not have any trouble sleeping because of it. Sleep management was not necessary as part of his treatment program.

Case 59: She had trouble sleeping because of her tinnitus. She bought a tabletop sound machine that played white noise. Her partner didn't like the sound, so she also used a pillow with a flat speaker inside that was compatible with her sound machine. She could hear the sound when her head was on her pillow, but her partner didn't hear the sound. She found she slept better when her tinnitus didn't sound so noticeable in the quiet bedroom.

Case 60: He had severe tinnitus. He went to an audiologist with specialized training in Tinnitus Retraining Therapy for counselling and sound therapy. The sound therapy included using white noise through a tabletop sound machine while sleeping. He found that using one device made it seem like the sound was coming too much from one direction. He ended up using two devices on either side of the bed so that the sound was more "stereo". He found this helped him sleep significantly better. He also used prescription drugs on a short-term basis (approximately 3 months) to help improve his sleep patterns as he got used to the sound enrichment. Over time his doctor helped him phase out the medication. He ended up only using sleep drugs for flare-ups.

Case 61: She had moderate tinnitus, and noticed sleep difficulties. She began exercising more regularly, and cut out tea and coffee in the evening. While sleeping, she used a tabletop sound machine that was set to relaxation sounds. She also tried deep breathing before falling asleep. Overall, these approaches helped her sleep better.

Case 62: He had severe tinnitus, and found a clinic offering tinnitus music therapy. He used his custom music device for day and night sound enrichment as recommended by his care provider. Over time, he noticed good improvement in his sleep and coping abilities.

Case 63: She had normal hearing and reported tinnitus distress during the day and when trying to fall asleep. She refused to use sound enrichment or any other treatment approach (e.g. mind enrichment, medication, etc.). She continued to have difficulty sleeping. None of the options suggested by the care provider were acceptable. Her care provider recommended she contact them in future if she decided to try appropriate treatment.

Case 64: He was only distressed by his tinnitus at bedtime. When he took his hearing aids out, his tinnitus became really noticeable making it hard for him to sleep. He discussed options with his audiologist. He had a bedroom fan that made a comfortable white noise type sound. He began turning it on regularly each night, and found the fan helped make his tinnitus less noticeable. He decided to order a white noise tabletop sound machine through his audiologist for year round use. At bedtime he also listened to music with the radio set to turn off automatically after enough time for him to fall asleep. Eventually he noticed that even though he could still hear his tinnitus when he took out his hearing aids, it didn't bother him any more.

Case 65: She had tinnitus, and tried various strategies to sleep better including white noise sound enrichment. She kept having sleep difficulties. She was referred to a sleep clinic, and was diagnosed with a sleep disorder. Treatment options were reviewed, and she decided to get a dental appliance. Once she started wearing it regularly, she noticed a significant improvement in her sleep.

Case 66: He had sound sensitivity and sleep difficulties. There were no specialized treatment clinics in his local area. He went to a counselling specialist to learn strategies to sleep better (e.g. distraction, relaxation, imagery, etc.). His sleep improved as he added techniques into his daily bedtime routine.

Case 67: He had tinnitus and slept poorly. He thought his tinnitus was really disturbing his sleep. He was having a lot of problems with his jaw, and talked to his dentist about it. They recommended treatment including wearing an appliance at night to help him stop grinding his teeth. After several months, his jaw began to feel better. His sleep partner noticed he made a lot of noise while sleeping. His doctor referred him to a sleep clinic, and he was diagnosed and treated for a sleep disorder.

Case 68: She used earplugs to sleep at night, and began noticing tinnitus. Over time, she began to notice the tinnitus getting so loud that it made it hard for her to sleep at all. She began using earplugs during the day as well to try to stop her tinnitus from getting worse. She saw an audiologist offering Progressive Tinnitus Management who strongly recommended that she stop using hearing protection for sleep or for daytime when there was no hazardous noise around. Sleep sound enrichment was recommended instead. She tried various sound types, and ended up making a custom digital recording of a relaxing sound that she preferred. She could set it to run all night through a bedside speaker. With time, she began sleeping better. Hearing protection management was also recommended to help her phase out her unhelpful habit of using hearing protection for everyday sound.

HEARING PROTECTION
MANAGEMENT

Hear today. Hear tomorrow. Christine Harrison,
Occupational Audiologist.

People with tinnitus and sound sensitivity may worry about hearing loss and hearing changes from noise. People often notice that loud sounds or noisy environments make their tinnitus seem worse. People with sound sensitivity may notice sounds or environments seem uncomfortably loud to them, but the noise doesn't bother other people. It is not always possible to turn down the volume or walk away from noise in our environment. So people may start to wear hearing protection (earplugs or earmuffs) to limit the sound getting to their ears. The idea is to stop their hearing loss, tinnitus or sound sensitivity from getting worse.

When sound is a potential noise hazard to the ears, then using appropriate hearing protection is an excellent strategy. The most common problem is overprotection. Overprotection is when a person wears hearing protection with too much sound reduction for their noise exposure. People may use hearing protection that blocks out as much sound as possible regardless of the amount of noise they are in, or they protect their ears all the time just in case a loud sound happens. It is important to be aware that overprotection makes it hard to hear voices or warning signals, especially for anyone with hearing loss. Overprotection can also make sound sensitivity and tinnitus worse.

The solution is not to wear hearing protection unless you need to. When you do need to wear hearing protection, do not over protect your ears by blocking out too much sound. Hearing protection is available that lowers the volume safely without overprotecting. Just as sunglasses are now available that automatically adjust for the brightness around you, there is also hearing protection available that adjusts for the loudness around you. This chapter discusses noise and noise hazards. It also describes hearing protection options appropriate for the specific needs of people with hearing loss, tinnitus and/or sound sensitivity.

NOISE

Noise is often defined as an unpleasant or loud sound. Noise can be unpleasantly loud without being hazardous to the ears, or noise can be unpleasantly loud and a noise hazard. Many loud sounds that are annoying, interfere with conversations, or aggravate tinnitus or sound sensitivity are still not hazardously noisy. Noise hazard depends on two factors: sound loudness and length of exposure. For a sound to be hazardously noisy, there must be sufficient intensity or sound power to cause ear damage. The duration or length of time a person is exposed to a sound also contributes to whether a sound is a hazardous or not. Extremely loud sounds can be hazardous with a short length of exposure. But many very loud sounds are not hazardous unless a person has a lengthy exposure regularly over a period of years.

Sound Intensity

plus Length of Exposure

equals NOISE HAZARD

As discussed in the chapter on How We Hear, sound loudness or intensity is measured in decibels (dB). The larger the dB value, the more intense the sound is. Noise most hazardous to human ears is measured in dBA. Doing noise measurement and analysis to check on whether noise is hazardous or not is a very complex process best left to professionals (e.g. acoustical engineers, occupational safety and health experts, etc). This chapter has very basic simple descriptions of the most common types of noise people come across in their work, recreation or everyday activities.

CHRONIC NOISE HAZARD

Chronic noise hazard is intense sound exposure that occurs regularly over time. It most commonly happens when people are exposed day after day to work or military noise. It is generally accepted that sounds of 85 dBA or greater have potential to cause permanent hearing damage after years of exposure. As a general rule of thumb if you have to shout to be heard by somebody standing 3 feet away, then the noise could be hazardously loud. Sounds in the 85 dBA range include a blender (e.g. mixing up a smoothie). Usually people wouldn't listen to a blender all day every day. So occasional short exposure would not cause any hearing loss. It is with long hours of repeated exposure over a number of years that permanent hearing damage can happen.

Imagine a lovely grassy lawn. Someone starts walking across the grass the same way every day. The grass will be crumpled, but will spring back up in between times. Eventually if the grass is walked over repeatedly all day long for day after day, it will wear down a path. The grass will be tramped down and not grow back. Similarly, the ear system can handle some noise occasionally. But if the noise happens repeatedly over time, then a path of damage gets worn down in the system. Permanent damage happens if the ear is overworked for too long.

In affected workers, research shows that it takes approximately 10 years of regular daily exposure to 85 dBA hazardous noise for a mild high frequency hearing loss to develop. The more intense the exposure, the faster and greater the hearing loss. Hearing loss and tinnitus from a chronic noise hazard are often temporary at first. For example, people may notice tinnitus and/or muffled hearing after a work shift but then it is gone by the next morning. This is sometimes called early warning tinnitus and temporary hearing shift.

Early warning tinnitus is an early warning sign that repeated exposure to the same noise without hearing protection could lead to permanent tinnitus and hearing loss. In the past it was sometimes referred to as "disco tinnitus" since people would experience ringing in their ears (and sometimes muffled hearing) after spending time in noisy situations such as a nightclub. Thankfully disco is dead, and "early warning tinnitus" is a preferred term. This tinnitus settles down with time away from noise as the ear recovers. However, with repeated exposure this tinnitus can become permanent or constant.

Temporary hearing shift (also called temporary threshold shift in the scientific literature) is a short term hearing change noticed as muffled or impaired hearing after exposure to noise. This temporary hearing shift happens after unprotected exposure then gradually recovers over time. If there is repeated exposure without hearing protection, then permanent hearing loss can develop. Temporary hearing shift often happens along with early warning tinnitus.

Over time, chronic hazardous noise can damage unprotected hearing structures inside the inner ear causing permanent noise-induced hearing loss. People with noise-induced hearing loss may also develop constant tinnitus. Chronic hazardous noise typically causes a pattern of high pitch sensorineural hearing loss in both ears with good hearing in the low to mid pitches. Sometimes noise related loss has a high pitch notched pattern although a notched pattern can also be due to various other causes. Past noise does not trigger a future hearing loss. Once you are away from noise, hearing does not keep changing from past noise. Many people with high pitch hearing loss have never been exposed to hazardous noise. Since many factors can cause high pitch sensorineural hearing loss (including aging), there must be a history of sufficient hazardous noise exposure to cause hearing loss before a hearing loss can be considered noise related.

Chronic noise hazard is most commonly from occupational noise, where a person is exposed repeatedly at work without protection on a regular daily basis over a number of years. Some examples of hazardous occupational noise sources may include mills, factories, manufacturing plants, shipyards, construction, carpentry, heavy equipment or truck operation, fish or tug boats, logging, forestry, mining, landscaping, aviation, bands or orchestras. Military exposure can also be a chronic noise hazard depending on the activities involved.

There are various agencies in different countries that have regulations and guidelines on workplace noise and hearing loss prevention. These may include provincial and territorial Workers' Compensation Boards in Canada, the National Institute for Occupational Safety and Health (NIOSH) or the Occupational Safety and Health Administration (OSHA) in the United States of America, the European Agency for Safety and Health at Work (EU-OSHA), the Australian Safety and Compensation Council (ASCC), etc. Employers typically have responsibilities to reduce noise (e.g. through engineering controls), inform workers of noise hazard areas, and to provide hearing protection.

Various sources of recreational noise can also be a chronic noise hazard if loud exposure happens regularly over time. Examples of potentially hazardous recreational noise or noise environments include music, personal music systems, lawn mowing (gas mower), power tools, saws, fitness classes, truck and tractor pulls, amusement parks, airplanes or air shows, model air plane flying, arcade games, nightclubs, bands, concerts, snowmobiles, motorcycles, All Terrain Vehicles (quads), and professional sporting events (e.g. hockey, football, wrestling).

You don't need exact noise measurements to protect your ears appropriately from noise. If you are repeatedly in a noise hazard (e.g. going to work everyday, cutting the lawn once a week with a gas mower, woodworking as a hobby, or using season tickets to your favourite football team), then wear appropriate hearing protection. If you are in loud noise occasionally (e.g. using a snowmobile a few days a month over the winter; going to an air show once a year), then the overall length of noise exposure is not sufficient to cause permanent hearing damage. But you could still notice muffled hearing, aggravated tinnitus, or discomfort from the sound. Some people have even had permanent tinnitus start after only one exposure to a loud activity. So it is always recommended you use hearing protection whenever you are around loud sound. Just make sure that you pick hearing protection that is appropriate for people with hearing loss, tinnitus or sound sensitivity.

ACUTE NOISE HAZARD

Acute noise hazard may be present for short (e.g. less than 60 seconds) extremely high intensity sound exposure. Acoustic trauma refers to the effects of one or a few exposures to very high levels of sound. If the sound power is intense enough, a brief exposure can cause immediate tinnitus and hearing loss. One might consider this a "sound bruise" to the ear. Just as regular bruises heal, hearing loss and tinnitus associated with a single ear "bruise" is usually temporary at first and gradually recovers over time. It is uncommon for a single encounter with an acute noise hazard to cause permanent hearing loss.

It usually takes an extreme intensity sound (e.g. blast or explosion) to cause permanent acute noise-induced hearing loss. When acute noise trauma happens, the ear system is stretched beyond its limits. In these cases, the ear has had a major blow not just a "bruise". Depending on the ear closest to the event, the trauma may cause hearing loss in one ear or worse in one ear. Any hearing loss is usually at the same frequency range as the traumatic sound. If inner ear damage happens with an extremely intense one time exposure (e.g. blast or explosion), the exposure may also cause middle ear damage (e.g. ruptured ear drum, damaged middle ear bones) along with permanent inner ear hearing loss. There can be partial or full hearing recovery within the first 6 to 12 months after the event. Any tinnitus may also fully or partially settle down over time.

If single acoustic trauma events become repeated (e.g. from unprotected gunfire exposure), then over time there can be permanent hearing loss and tinnitus. Imagine being hit and bruised over and over again on the same spot. The ear structures can't take repeated hits. Eventually permanent ear damage will happen. For gunfire exposure, there is a typical pattern of high pitch sensorineural hearing loss in both ears, but worse in one ear if weapons are fired from the shoulder. The opposite ear to the shoulder supporting a rifle or shotgun in firing position is actually closer or more open to the sound impact. For example, for right shoulder shooters, the worst hearing loss is in the left ear.

People with tinnitus or sound sensitivity often worry about loud bangs or sounds that occasionally happen as they go through their daily activities. It is important to remember that these types of occasional loud sounds are not an acute noise hazard. Acoustic trauma comes with extreme sound power. Hunting or gunfire exposure is probably the most significant acute noise hazard. Explosions, bomb blasts, release of high pressure valves, faulty equipment or other intense sound events may also cause acoustic trauma. In workplace settings, acute noise is most commonly caused by accidents or incidents where sudden extreme unexpected noise occurs. Military exposure (especially wartime) is also a common acute noise hazard.

Since acute noise hazards are typically accidental and unexpected, people usually aren't wearing hearing protection. Gunfire exposure (e.g. hunting, military) is a significant exception because people know they will be exposed to noise from gunfire. It is strongly recommended people use appropriate hearing protection for gunfire exposure since any related hearing loss is preventable. When a person works in a chronic noise hazard and is using hearing protection, then that hearing protection will also give some protection against any accidental acute noise hazard. If people with sound sensitivity (or tinnitus) use hearing protection for occasional loud noise, they should make sure they choose appropriate hearing protection.

MUSIC HAZARD

Noise is usually defined as unwanted sound. Music is a wanted sound. But if music is listened to very loudly and repeatedly, then there is the same risk of permanent hearing loss and tinnitus as there is for any other hazardous noise exposure. Children and adults are affected similarly. Noise is noise. Ears are ears. Both music and noise can cause similar high frequency permanent hearing loss with repeated exposure over time. When this hearing loss is from music, it is called music-induced hearing loss. This type of hearing loss can be associated with people who regularly use personal music devices, musicians, and people who regularly go to nightclubs or loud concerts. Any type of music from rock, blues, jazz or classical can be a hazard. It is important to remember that just like with any other noise hazard, music hazard depends on the volume (sound intensity) and listening time (length of exposure). Some people have had permanent tinnitus start after only one exposure to loud music (e.g. concert or nightclub).

Personal music players have led to a huge increase in the amount of time daily that people listen to music. Batteries can now last for hours and devices can store hundreds of songs. This can be helpful for sound enrichment as long as only soft to moderate sound loudness is used (no more than half volume at most). Otherwise listening to loud music for extended periods of time can increase risk of music-induced hearing loss. There are headphones available with built-in sound limiters so music can't exceed hazardous levels. Some devices also have volume limiters that can be locked so the volume control can't be turned above a set level. Headphones or earphones with noise cancellation or "isolation" features are also available to reduce background noise so you don't have to turn the music up as loud to hear it.

Hearing protection should be used for other music hazards (e.g. playing in a band, going to a concert). People are often very resistant to the thought of using hearing protection for music. But there is high fidelity hearing protection available that is designed specifically for music lovers and musicians from rock bands to orchestras. It has a filter that lowers sound volume without distortion or echo. This specialized hearing protection is very appropriate for people with hearing loss, tinnitus or sound sensitivity who want to enjoy music safely. Other products and devices are also available to help lower music exposure for musicians. Information is available through various musician related groups and Websites.

EVERYDAY NOISE

As discussed in the chapter on Sound Enrichment, it is well established that people with tinnitus should try to surround themselves with pleasant or neutral sound. However, in daily life it is only natural that some of the time there will be noisy sound in our environment. People (especially with tinnitus or sound sensitivity) tend to think any loud unpleasant noise is dangerous to their ears.

Sound can be loud enough to be annoying or interfere with conversations or activities and still not be hazardously loud.

Another undesirable effect is that loud sound can be uncomfortable for people with sound sensitivity. Louder noise or sound can also make tinnitus worse for some people. The tinnitus becomes worse during or after they are in noisy environments. The tinnitus then settles back down after the person is away from noise. It may sometimes take hours (or longer) after returning to quieter environments for the tinnitus to settle. It is easy to confuse this with early warning tinnitus. But sound does not have to be hazardous to be uncomfortable or aggravate tinnitus. This effect can be caused by various everyday sounds (e.g. driving in the car with the window open, going to a busy restaurant, etc.). It is the nature of the beast.

Often people incorrectly think a noise must be hazardous if it interferes with communication, sounds uncomfortable, or bothers their tinnitus or sound sensitivity. They may start to have worry, anxiety, annoyance, fear and anger over whether they are exposing themselves to a noise hazard. As discussed in the chapter on How We Hear Tinnitus, these emotional reactions can increase sensitivity or activity within the hearing system. This has a negative effect on sound sensitivity and tinnitus distress. While most people wouldn't think of using hearing protection for everyday noise, some people with tinnitus or sound sensitivity may start using ear protection in their everyday life when they find the world around them too loud. Hearing protection is not generally recommended for regular everyday sound. But when a person can't get by without it, then treatment should involve using appropriate hearing protection. With treatment, people with tinnitus or sound sensitivity may be able to gradually wean off hearing protection for everyday noise over time. If not, the goal is to only use hearing protection appropriate for tinnitus or sound sensitivity.

HEARING PROTECTION

Hearing protection that is appropriate for people in general is not necessarily appropriate for people with hearing loss, tinnitus and/or sound sensitivity. Hearing protection are devices like earplugs or earmuffs that are worn in or over the ears. They are designed to lower the loudness of hazardous environmental sound to non-hazardous levels. Essentially hearing protection gives you a hearing loss (or increases your existing hearing loss) so that you can't hear as well. An audiologist or tinnitus specialist can help guide people in selecting appropriate hearing protection.

Hearing protection comes in various styles of earplugs and earmuffs. Earplugs stop noise by sealing or blocking off the ear canal. They come in three main styles: compressible, reusable, and reusable canal cap. Compressible earplugs are often made of foam, sponge, or glass down. They are squeezed or rolled thinner, and then inserted into the ear canal where they expand to fill and block it off. Limited sizes are available. Reusable earplugs are made of vinyl or silicone. They may be custom molded to fit a person's ears or be pre-molded plastic with flanges to fit different sized ear canals. Reusable canal cap earplugs are inserted into the ear canal or cover the ear canal opening. A plastic or metal band connects the earplugs. The band can be worn in various positions (e.g. over the head, under the chin). Sometimes the band makes an unpleasant noise if it is rubbed or knocked.

Earmuffs have cups with a hard shell that reflects sound away from the ear, and a sound absorbent cuff to snugly fit around your ear and stop sound from leaking in. A plastic or metal headband connects the cups. They come in different headband styles including over the head, behind the neck, or beneath the chin. Hardhat mounting is also available with many earmuff models. Because ears come in so many sizes and shapes, earmuffs also come in different sizes and shapes depending on the manufacturer. They should fit close to your head with no gaps, and feel comfortable over time. Earmuffs should not be modified (e.g. don't drill holes into the cups for better air circulation and don't alter them to allow music reception). User modifications will destroy the protection available.

If you want to safely listen to music while you are in hazardous noise, some manufacturers offer earmuff style hearing protection with built-in music capability. This hearing protection screens out hazardous noise while playing music limited to a safe loudness inside the earmuffs. People working in hazardously noisy repetitive or monotonous work environments often use this type of hearing protection. Some models have built-in AM/FM radios. Other models allow you to plug in a personal music listening system.

Hearing protection lasts different amounts of time depending on the style as well as how they are cared for. Compressible earplugs are usually used once and then discarded (although some people re-use them a few times if they don't get dirty). With regular use, reusable pre-formed earplugs last approximately 6 to 12 months. They should not be used if they lose their pre-formed shape, the plastic begins to deteriorate, or they can't be wiped clean. Reusable custom earplugs last approximately 3 to 4 years. They can be wiped clean, so they are reusable until the material starts to harden or deteriorate. Reusable canal cap earplugs last approximately 6 to 12 months. They are reusable until the band loses its spring or tension, they lose their pre-formed shape, the material begins to deteriorate, or they can't be cleaned properly. Earmuffs will last about 4 to 5 years, but the soft sound absorbent cuff or pad (the part that sits next to your skin) should be replaced approximately once a year when the plastic deteriorates or the pad loses it's cushioning.

Hearing protection is offered in various styles since what works best for one person's needs may not be appropriate for somebody else. Some people have a preference for earmuffs over earplugs. Some people have better fit and greater comfort with an earplug than an earmuff depending on head size or shape, ear canal size or shape, or finger dexterity (e.g. ability to insert a plug). Other considerations when selecting the style include use of eyeglasses (earmuffs may be uncomfortable and not seal properly around the ear), excess earwax or middle ear problems (should not wear earplugs), use of other personal protective equipment (e.g. hardhats, safety glasses, welding gear, etc.). Climate can also make a difference. If people are in hot and/or humid noisy environments, then earplugs may be more comfortable and help minimize skin irritation. Some people who work outside switch from earplugs in summer to earmuffs in winter.

People with hearing loss who usually use hearing aids can have difficulty with hearing protection. Hearing protection makes hearing worse. So some people may still wear hearing aids or choose earmuffs to go over top of the hearing aids when they are in a noise hazard environment. The problem is that hearing aids and very loud noise don't go together. If turned off, hearing aids are not a hearing protector. If turned on, hearing aids are not designed to block out sound enough to protect against hazardous noise. It can also be hot and humid underneath an earmuff, which is not good for hearing aid electronics. People with hearing loss should never wear their hearing aids while in hazardous noise environments (either alone or under earmuff style hearing protection). There are appropriate hearing protection options available.

People should choose a hearing protection style that fits well and feels comfortable. In addition to considering comfort, earplugs and earmuffs come with various features. It is essential for people with hearing loss, tinnitus or sound sensitivity to choose features that offer appropriate protection for their individual needs. Four main features to consider include amount of sound reduction, pattern of sound reduction, electronic sound reduction, and communication capability.

AMOUNT OF SOUND REDUCTION

Hearing protection comes in different grades or classes depending on the noise reduction rating (NRR). The noise reduction rating (in dB) is included on the hearing protection label or packaging. It indicates how much the hearing protector will reduce sound but only if it fits properly and is worn the whole time a person is in a noise hazard. The higher the NRR, the more sound can be blocked out. Double or dual protection of earmuffs plus earplugs worn together has very high sound reduction. Class A, Grade 3 or Grade 4 hearing protection has high sound reduction. Class B or Grade 2 hearing protection has moderate sound reduction. Class C or Grade 1 hearing protection has low sound reduction. A noise reduction rating of >24 dB gives high sound reduction. A noise reduction rating of ≤24 dB would give low to moderate sound reduction.

The higher the noise hazard, the higher the amount of sound reduction (NRR) recommended. Examples of extremely high noise hazard environments include running chainsaws or jackhammers, underground mining, flight deck personnel (e.g. for military jets), etc. In these high noise environments, high sound reduction hearing protection is typically required and should be used to protect hearing. Sometimes people working in extreme noise will even need to "double-up" or wear earplugs underneath their earmuffs in order to provide maximum sound reduction. Double or dual protection is often used in environments where verbal communication would be impossible and warning signals would be inaudible because of the high intensity of the surrounding noise. Maximum protection should only be used for this extreme noise power.

Most people are familiar with high sound reduction hearing protection. This traditional hearing protection includes compressible earplugs, some reusable earplugs or canal caps, reusable custom molded solid earplugs, and heavy solid earmuffs. This is mainly because people have adopted a "more is better" approach, trying to block out as much sound as possible with hearing protection. People have assumed that higher sound reduction or the highest grade or class must mean the "best" protection. The problem is that even in many hazardously noisy environments high sound reduction hearing protection blocks out too much sound. The result is too much simulated hearing loss that makes it hard to hear speech, warning signals or necessary sounds.

People with tinnitus and/or sound sensitivity should certainly consider maximum protection when in extreme noise. If you are planning on cutting your winter firewood with a chainsaw, mowing the lawn with a gas mower, or doing other very high noise activities then high sound reduction hearing protection is fine to use. But it is common to see people with tinnitus and sound sensitivity select the highest available sound reduction they can find in hearing protection regardless of the amount of noise. They will often choose high sound reduction protection for work noise, recreational noise, or even noise from everyday activities. Audiologists or tinnitus specialists also see people with tinnitus or sound sensitivity who double-up by using earplugs and earmuffs together to protect their ears. Most use double protection even though they are not in extreme noise environments. They mistakenly think it is better for their ears to block out as much sound as possible on a routine everyday basis. Unfortunately, using high protection or high double protection when not needed can result in overprotection that actually makes tinnitus and sound sensitivity worse.

Hearing protection with more moderate sound reduction is available (NRR ≤24 dB). This moderate reduction is an appropriate choice to give safe protection without overprotecting the ears. Just like you don't want sunglasses that darken so much it is too hard to see, you don't want hearing protection that blocks so much sound that it is too hard to hear what you still need to. Research shows that a moderate sound reducing hearing protection is appropriate even for many hazardously noisy work environments. Moderate sound reduction hearing protection cuts out less sound or gives less simulated hearing loss. A person wearing moderate sound reduction protection can hear necessary speech or sounds better while still protecting their hearing. Moderate sound reduction hearing protection is available in reusable earplugs or canal caps as well as earmuff styles. If they are not in extreme noise, people with tinnitus or sound sensitivity should consider hearing protection with moderate sound reduction.

PATTERN OF SOUND REDUCTION

Another feature to consider with hearing protection is the pattern of sound reduction. In addition to a high amount of sound reduction, traditional hearing protection also gives a high frequency pattern of sound reduction. Very simply, this is because high frequencies reflect the most off traditional earplugs or earmuffs. You may have noticed a similar effect if you have ever lived in an apartment next to a neighbour who liked playing loud music. The high frequencies are blocked or reflected better by walls, so you end up hearing the muffled thumping bass coming through. The problem with traditional high frequency sound reduction hearing protection is that you get a similar muffled sound. The simulated hearing loss from this hearing protection is greatest in the high frequency range.

Hearing protection with this high frequency pattern can distort sound and impair communication just like having any type of high frequency hearing loss. This may aggravate tinnitus and sound sensitivity, as well as further impair hearing for people with underlying hearing loss. It makes it that much harder to hear necessary speech, warning signals or environmental sounds. When a person has to keep straining to hear, it can lead to anxiety, stress and fatigue, which is not good for anyone, but particularly for people with tinnitus or sound sensitivity. See chapter on Hearing Loss Management for more information on the negative effects of "straining to hear". This effect can happen from any hearing loss including a "hearing protection loss". It is important to protect hearing while minimizing any sound distortion present.

An appropriate alternative for people with hearing loss, tinnitus or sound sensitivity is to select hearing protection with a flat or uniform pattern of sound reduction. This type of hearing protection has filters to reduce sound equally at all pitches or frequencies. The effect is like turning down the volume. A flat pattern of sound reduction prevents sound distortion and keeps speech and other sounds clear and unmuffled. This type of hearing protection dates back to the 1970's when musicians in music hazards refused to wear hearing protection because it made the music sound distorted. This led to the Musician's™ flat pattern custom molded filtered earplugs that were designed to make sound heard through these earplugs have good clarity but just be quieter. Hearing protection with a flat pattern is often referred to as high fidelity. This type of hearing protection is available in reusable filtered earplugs (pre-molded or custom) and filtered earmuffs. As well as being used for protection from hazardous noise, the earplug styles can be useful as part of treatment for people with tinnitus or sound sensitivity that want protection from occasional or intermittent uncomfortably loud non-hazardous everyday sounds.

ELECTRONIC SOUND REDUCTION

The need for electronic sound reduction should also be considered when selecting hearing protection. Traditional hearing protection gives the same amount of sound reduction as long as it is worn no matter how loud the surrounding sound is. If someone is working or playing in hazardous noise that is constant over time, then constant sound reduction is fine. But many people work or play where the noise hazard varies in loudness. In these situations, it is not appropriate to use traditional constant protection. An appropriate option for people with hearing loss, tinnitus or sound sensitivity is to use electronic protection that automatically adjusts for the sound loudness. This is particularly important to avoid overprotection.

Electronic hearing protection is currently only available in earmuff style given the space required for the electronics and batteries. Electronic earmuffs were originally designed for military and police to allow them to hear quiet sounds (e.g. whispering or rustling of enemies or suspects) but then instantly protect if there was any sudden loud sound (e.g. gunfire). They work so successfully that they have become popular for various work and recreational noise hazards. Electronic earmuffs have a knob or button to turn them on. When turned on, a microphone picks up sound outside the earmuff. The electronics then measure the sound level and automatically adjust as needed. Soft to moderate sounds are allowed in and may be boosted or amplified in volume, while loud sounds are safely reduced. When turned off, the muffs reduce sound similarly to traditional earmuffs.

Some electronic hearing protection has a volume control so the wearer can adjust the volume setting. Voices and equipment warning signals are characteristically much softer than the surrounding noise hazard. This type of hearing protection allows safe built-in volume adjustments to make it much easier to hear speech, equipment, or warning sounds. This feature is particularly helpful for people with hearing loss since it is like having a safe built-in hearing aid within the hearing protection. When the sound reaching the inside of the earmuff is loud to hazardously loud, the electronics reduce the sound safely and do not allow further amplification or volume increase.

Some manufacturers offer electronic earmuffs with a "push to talk" feature instead of a volume control. When off, the muffs reduce all sound. But when turned on, soft to moderate sounds (e.g. voices) are amplified or boosted safely while loud sounds are safely reduced. The increased safe volume only stays on for a few minutes. The idea is a person can have a brief conversation while working in noise (e.g. with a co-worker or supervisor) and then the hearing protection goes back to its usual constant sound reduction when no communication is happening.

Electronic hearing protection is available in monaural (one external microphone) and stereo (two external microphones). People who need to locate sound sources while in a noise hazard should use the stereo version. With electronic hearing protection people don't need to lift off their hearing protector to talk or hear important sounds, so they do a much better job of protecting their hearing from noise hazards. Electronic hearing protection also helps people with hearing loss more easily communicate and hear any necessary machine or warning signals while still protecting their hearing. Some models are also available with built-in communication systems.

COMMUNICATION SYSTEMS

Some people working in noise hazards need to use communication systems like one or two way radios or other communication devices. Hearing protection is available that allows input directly from communication systems. The connection can be hands-free, hard-wire or wireless. This type of hearing protection is particularly helpful for people with hearing loss who also need to use communication systems while working in a noise hazard. The communication system capability is often an available option with electronic hearing protection. Reusable custom molded solid earplugs can also be ordered with communication system plug in capability although they can't give any boost or amplification for soft to moderate sounds like electronic earmuffs can.

NOISE CANCELLATION

Some people wonder why they can't use hearing protection that just cancels out the noise around them. Noise cancellation hearing protection and devices are available, but this electronic technology is mainly useful for certain specific noise hazard environments. However, this technology is also available to reduce non-hazardous background noise. Many airplane passengers use this type of noise cancellation device to reduce aircraft cabin noise. These devices can make flying in an airplane a much more easy and comfortable listening environment. They can be very helpful when people with hearing loss, tinnitus and/or sound sensitivity are travelling by plane. Various electronic noise cancellation headphones and earpieces are available. Noise cancellation systems are often available from stores or companies offering travel or relaxation related products. Sound quality can vary so it is wise to comparison shop. Some people also use noise cancellation devices in other everyday environments where they want to increase listening comfort by reducing ambient background noise.

SLEEP PROTECTION

Hearing protection is not recommended for sleep. See the chapter on Sleep Management. People with distressing tinnitus or sound sensitivity should always try to use sound enrichment set at a comfortable loudness for sleep. Using hearing protection to sleep can and will make tinnitus and sound sensitivity worse. Even if you are a shift worker, it is much better to use comfortable moderate relaxation sound to help screen out environmental sounds while sleeping than to use hearing protection. Hearing protection for sleep should only be considered on an occasional short-term "emergency" basis (e.g. you happen to be traveling or away from home and don't have any sound enrichment devices available, and noisy neighbours are keeping you awake). The goal is to get back to your usual sleep sound enrichment routine as soon as possible.

SOUND SENSITIVITY

Almost half of people with tinnitus also have sound sensitivity. Often people with severe sound sensitivity avoid sound to the extent of overprotecting their ears with earplugs and/or earmuffs when they are not around hazardous noise. Research shows that this overprotection makes sound sensitivity (and tinnitus) worse. If you wear hearing protection inappropriately, then your ears will become more sensitive. The good news is that sound sensitivity can be reversed through treatment. Along with counselling therapy, treatment typically includes using sound enrichment (including in-ear sound generators or combination instruments if recommended) and using hearing protection appropriately.

Sound sensitivity is treatable. It just takes time. Each person in treatment needs to go at his or her own pace. Over a period of months, your audiologist or sound sensitivity treatment provider (often a tinnitus specialist or Tinnitus/ Auditory Retraining Therapy specialist) can guide you through a sound sensitivity treatment plan that is customized for you. If a person has been overprotecting their ears with hearing protection, then part of the treatment plan should include hearing protection management.

People with sound sensitivity often wear single or double traditional hearing protection with constant high sound reduction. Unless you are in an extreme noise hazard (where everybody is required to wear high sound reduction or double hearing protection), then it is highly likely overprotection is happening. The problem is that sound sensitive people find it extremely difficult to change or stop their use of ear protectors. Their ears have gotten used to the reduced sound input. It can be a challenge to re-introduce more sound. Discomfort or sensitivity can happen when the ears process more sound, just like muscles can hurt if we exercise after a period of low activity. Hearing protection management typically involves a very gradual change over from the constant high sound reduction traditional protection to more appropriate options. For everyday noise, the use of any hearing protection may eventually be phased out completely if possible.

I can't emphasize enough that sound sensitivity treatment must be individually customized while the person being treated is guided and supported through the process. People with hearing loss or tinnitus alone can switch hearing protection with no discomfort (and usually a big increase in comfort). A sudden change in hearing protection is often unsuccessful for people with sound sensitivity since they need to get used to how things should sound through their appropriate safe hearing protection. A gradual change in combination with regular counselling and guidance to discuss any concerns is usually most comfortable. If you work in hazardous noise, then your care provider can help guide you on any adjustments you need to make for work while you are going through treatment. The following examples are not intended to replace the advice of your audiologist or sound sensitivity treatment provider.

Sound Sensitivity Example—Change to Electronic Earmuffs:
A person is wearing traditional high sound reduction earmuffs plus foam earplugs in a work noise hazard although this amount of sound reduction is not necessary or required in their place of employment. They are overprotecting their ears. Their sound sensitivity care provider has recommended electronic earmuffs. First they may gradually phase out use of the foam earplugs by spending more and more time only using the traditional earmuffs alone. Once they are just using the earmuffs, then they could phase out the traditional earmuffs by gradually switching to wearing electronic earmuffs but used turned off (to give constant sound reduction). Then they could start phasing in the automatic capability by wearing the electronic earmuffs turned on when they need to hear voices or equipment sounds or for at last 5 to 15 minutes per shift. The goal could be to eventually try to wear the earmuffs turned on to a comfortable volume for as much of the shift as possible to keep the ears "exercised" with safe soft to moderate sound (e.g. very gradually increase amount of time turned on each shift even if only by 15 minutes over a work week).

A different person in the same circumstances might find it easier to first phase out use of the traditional earmuffs. They could gradually switch over to using the electronic earmuffs turned off over top of the foam earplugs. Then phase out use of the foam earplugs. Then phase in wearing the electronic earmuffs turned on to a comfortable volume when they need to hear voices or equipment sounds or for at last 5 to 15 minutes per shift. Again the goal could be to very gradually work up to wearing the earmuffs turned on to a comfortable volume for as much of each work shift as possible.

Sound Sensitivity Example—Change to Custom Molded Filtered Earplugs:

This person is wearing traditional high sound reduction earmuffs plus foam earplugs for their regular daily activities and work in non-hazardous noise. They are overprotecting their ears. Their sound sensitivity care provider has recommended custom molded filtered earplugs that will reduce loud sounds while keeping soft to moderate sounds and voices natural and easy to hear. First they could phase out the foam earplugs by gradually switching over to wearing custom molded filtered earplugs underneath the earmuffs. Then they could phase out the earmuffs by wearing them for less and less time each day as they worked towards only using the custom molded filtered earplugs.

A different person in the same circumstances might prefer to phase out using the earmuffs first. They could gradually wear the earmuffs less and less time each day working towards wearing only the foam earplugs. Then they could switch over to using the custom molded filtered earplugs instead of the foam plugs. They could phase out the foam earplugs by wearing them for less and less time each day and work up to just wearing the custom molded filtered earplugs.

HEARING PROTECTION PLAN

The best hearing protection is the one that you will wear for the entire time you're exposed to hazardous noise. Removing or lifting up hearing protection to talk or listen to signals even for brief periods in hazardous noise provides almost as little protection as no protection at all. Select an earmuff or earplug that is comfortable, allows you to hear necessary sounds or voices, and that you can wear consistently when you are in hazardous noise.

Table 10	
HEARING PROTECTION OPTIONS	
EARPLUG CHOICES INCLUDE:	
Moderate Reduction (NRR ≤24 dB)	• Pre-molded earplug • Canal cap or banded earplug
Flat Reduction ("high fidelity")	• Pre-molded filtered earplug • Custom molded filtered earplug
EARMUFF CHOICES INCLUDE:	
Moderate Reduction (NRR ≤24 dB)	• Earmuff
Flat Reduction ("high fidelity")	• Filtered earmuff
Safe Amplification	• Electronic earmuff • Electronic earmuff with communication capability

In most cases these options will give appropriate protection while giving a more natural sound quality and allowing easier communication. These features are certainly beneficial for people with hearing loss, tinnitus or sound sensitivity. In situations of extreme or high noise hazards, traditional hearing protection may still be necessary. An audiologist or tinnitus specialist can guide you in selecting the most appropriate hearing protection for your individual situation.

If you have sound sensitivity and need to use hearing protection for loud non-hazardous sound, it is usually more socially acceptable to use an earplug style. For example, people might wonder if you use earmuffs in a noisy restaurant when you are out to dinner with friends, but are unlikely to notice if you use filtered earplugs.

Cost can be a consideration. Pre-molded or canal cap earplugs cost less than custom molded filtered earplugs. Moderate sound reduction earmuffs or filtered earmuffs cost less than electronic earmuffs. Electronic earmuffs can still vary in cost. Some models (e.g. push to talk) cost as little as traditional earmuffs. Other types of electronic earmuffs are more expensive. But over time the benefits of appropriate hearing protection can far outweigh the cost for people with hearing loss, tinnitus or sound sensitivity. If you work in noise, often employers are required to supply hearing protection. This can include providing appropriate hearing protection to accommodate a person's hearing loss, tinnitus or sound sensitivity needs.

Ideally your audiologist or tinnitus/sound sensitivity treatment provider will give you a specific hearing protection recommendation. Custom molded filtered earplugs are usually available through your audiologist or treatment clinic. Pre-molded earplugs, canal caps or earmuffs are usually available through safety supply stores. Safety supply stores may not have appropriate models in stock but can order them in. Sometimes you will be able to try out options (e.g. electronic earmuffs from two different manufacturers) to see which sounds and feels best to you. There is also a lot of hearing protection information on the Internet on various manufacturer Websites. It can be helpful to browse manufacturer's catalogues for product descriptions and/or contact a manufacturer's representative to help find what you are looking for.

Other retailers (e.g. hardware or garden stores) may also carry hearing protection, although usually traditional high sound reduction earmuffs or compressible earplugs are the only choices offered. Some landscaping or woodworking related companies do have appropriate choices including electronic muffs with music capability offered at quite reasonable prices. The sound quality may not be as good as what is available through a safety supply store.

If you consistently use appropriate properly fitting hearing protection at all times when in hazardous noise, and your hearing keeps changing then the cause might not be noise. Hearing protection can only protect against noise related hearing changes. Don't forget that there are many causes of hearing loss that can affect people in general, including people who work or spend time in noisy environments. Noise can't be blamed for all hearing changes. Keep using appropriate hearing protection when in a noise hazard to prevent any noise related loss.

People with hearing loss, tinnitus and/or sound sensitivity may want to consider the following guidelines on hearing protection. These guidelines are not intended to replace the advice of your audiologist or tinnitus/sound sensitivity treatment provider.

- Don't use hearing protection for sleep. Use sound enrichment.

- When you are around loud noise or music, always wear appropriate hearing protection.

- Take advantage of appropriate earplug or earmuff options including moderate sound reduction, flat or "high fidelity" reduction, or electronic reduction with safe built-in amplification.

- Consider communication or music system capability if necessary.

- If you have hearing loss, never wear hearing aids in hazardous noise (either alone or under earmuffs). If you need to communicate or hear important sounds while in a noise hazard, try electronic earmuffs with safe built-in amplification.

- Only use traditional high sound reduction hearing protection or double-up (earplugs and earmuffs) if you are in an extreme noise hazard.

- If you are bothered by loud sounds or noise that are not considered hazardous, then filtered earplugs that keep things sounding natural while screening out loud sounds can be an appropriate option.

- Consider noise cancelling headphones or devices for increased listening comfort in certain non-hazardous everyday noise situations (e.g. travelling in an airplane).

It is well established that sound enrichment is extremely beneficial for people who have tinnitus and/or sound sensitivity. Using hearing protection gives a sound reduced instead of a sound enriched environment. So it is important to reduce sound only as much as necessary to protect hearing or to increase comfort. Since hearing protection greatly influences the amount of sound that is presented to the ears, it is very important for people with tinnitus and/or sound sensitivity to choose appropriate hearing protection. Whenever possible stay away from "traditional" high sound reduction distorting protectors that can overprotect the ears. Explore other appropriate options.

Author's Case: I have normal hearing and tinnitus. I also dislike loud sounds, which is a mild form of sound sensitivity. I remind myself that my ears are built to hear normal natural sounds from soft to loud. I don't regularly work in a noise hazard, but make occasional visits into noisy workplaces (e.g. sawmills, manufacturing plants, construction sites). At first I used traditional high sound reduction earmuffs or foam earplugs. Although they made the noise less loud, I found it really hard to have conversations with people while in the noisy areas. I switched to custom molded filtered earplugs. They helped cut the noise, but I could still hear well enough to understand speech clearer. I find these custom molded filtered earplugs are comfortable and also work well for any other occasional very loud noise I am in at home or play (e.g. lawnmower, saws, concerts, sports arenas, etc.). I also like to use noise cancellation headphones when I am travelling by airplane.

Case 69: She has tinnitus with normal hearing. She works in hazardous noise that is intermittent during her workday, but doesn't currently use hearing protection. She didn't like compressible earplugs because she couldn't squeeze them into her ear canals properly, they got dirty all the time, and she couldn't hear sounds or voices when she needed to. She didn't like earmuffs because they also blocked out too much and were too bulky. It was recommended she try pre-molded or custom molded filtered earplugs. Both these types of plugs would give moderate natural sound reduction. She could still hear soft to moderate sounds or voices while wearing them. They were easier to insert without getting dirty, and they didn't get in the way. She chose custom molded filtered earplugs since they were more cost effective over the long term.

Case 70: He has hearing loss and tinnitus. He can't hear his two-way radio at work even if he has his hearing aids on. He is also very worried he may damage his hearing more by wearing his hearing aids in a hazardously noisy work environment. Co-workers and supervisors are getting frustrated and angry at misunderstandings and mistakes made when he can't hear radioed information. It was recommended he try electronic earmuffs with radio plug-in, or custom molded earplugs: filtered in the left ear and solid with radio plug-in for the right ear (he preferred listening to the two way radio in his right ear).

Either option would allow him to hear radio communications better while also making it easier for him to hear warning signals or voices needed to work safely. He decided to use the electronic earmuffs with radio plug-in since they gave him some additional safe amplification for soft sounds and face-to-face conversations that wasn't available with the custom earplugs. Once he started using them, he received a lot of positive feedback at work on the improvement in his ability to accurately complete his job duties.

Case 71: He has tinnitus. He works in hazardous noise that varies up and down throughout his day. Every now and then he needs to talk to co-workers. In the past, he used hardhat mount high sound reduction earmuffs that he lifted off when he needed to talk. He has learned that this is almost as bad as not wearing any protection at all. He needs to find a hearing protector that he can wear continuously without lifting off. He prefers earmuffs. Possible earmuff options include moderate sound reduction, filtered, or electronic "push to talk". He liked how these options felt more lightweight and comfortable to wear than the traditional earmuffs. He tried out a filtered "high fidelity" model and a "push to talk" electronic model of earmuffs in the safety supply store to see which he liked best. He then ordered his selection in a hardhat mount.

Case 72: She has hearing loss and tinnitus. She works in constant hazardous noise. She currently uses high sound reduction earmuffs, but she finds she can't ear soft equipment or machinery noise she needs to do her work. She has no preference for a particular hearing protector style. It is recommended that she try moderate sound reduction pre-molded earplugs, earmuffs or electronic earmuffs. These options will help her hear softer sounds better while still protecting her hearing. The electronic muffs would give some added safe amplification at significantly higher cost. She tried out a moderate sound reduction earplug and then tried a moderate sound reduction earmuff, and found that each worked fine. She did not need any extra volume at work to compensate for her hearing loss once sound wasn't being blocked out so much. She decided on the moderate sound reduction protector that felt most comfortable.

Case 73: She has tinnitus. She plays in a loud band. She has tried foam earplugs, but they hurt her ears and distort the sound too much. It is recommended that she try custom molded filtered earplugs or Musician's™ earplugs. These will turn down the volume, but still help her hear music without distortion.

Case 74: He has tinnitus. He is a supervisor who usually works in an office. A couple of times a day he has to briefly go into noisy areas and talk to other workers. He hasn't been bothering with hearing protection since he finds it a hassle to put earplugs or earmuffs on for such short periods of time. It is recommended he try moderate sound reduction banded or canal cap earplugs. He can hang them around his neck when not wearing them. They are quick and easy to put on before he goes into a noisy area. He would still be able to hear well enough to talk to co-workers while wearing them. He is not worried about any potential annoying sound if the band gets rubbed or bumped.

Case 75: She has tinnitus. She works in hazardous noise in a very boring monotonous job. Some of her co-workers have slipped their personal listening device earpiece under their earmuffs so they can listen to music while working. She tried it. At the end of her shift, she noticed her tinnitus was worse. She realized she was turning the music up louder than the hazardous noise to hear it, which also put the music at a hazardously loud level. She was only increasing the overall noise hazard. She tried some earmuffs with safe built-in music reception. These worked well and helped pass the time at work.

Case 76: His family like going to air shows where there is a lot of noise from the aircraft flying overhead. They are noticing some muffled hearing and ringing in their ears after they leave. The family decides to get hearing protection. The younger children (under 12) get earmuffs specially designed smaller for kids. Nobody else wants an earmuff style, so they decide to get pre-molded filtered "high fidelity" earplugs. These plugs will cut out the noise sufficiently while still letting everyone hear conversations. Moderate sound reduction banded and custom molded filtered earplugs were also considered.

Case 77: She doesn't like how her tinnitus always gets worse after concerts. There is a band coming to town that she really likes so she bought tickets. The concert will be at a large arena. She finds foam earplugs uncomfortable, and they change how the music sounds. Since she goes to concerts a few times a year, she decides it is cost effective to get custom molded filtered earplugs or Musician's™ earplugs. These plugs will protect her hearing without distorting the music.

Case 78: She has tinnitus. She wants hearing protection to use while mowing the lawn. She just needs something to block out the noise. She looks at moderate and high sound reduction earmuffs and also compressible earplugs. Since she mows the lawn once a week for a few months a year, she decides earmuffs will be most cost effective. She gets the high sound reduction earmuffs to use only for the gas lawn mower or other power tools in the garden. This gives her high sound reduction, but just for a few hours each month.

Case 79: He has hearing loss and tinnitus. He has a woodworking shop in his garage. He likes to putter on various projects. He has high sound reduction earmuffs, but he finds them a bit bulky and warm. He decided to get moderate sound reduction banded earplugs that are lightweight and cooler to wear. He liked how they can hang around his neck, but he can quickly put them on before he hammers or runs power tools. After using them for a while, he didn't like how there was a funny noise when the band got bumped. He switched to moderate sound reduction "behind the neck" style earmuffs.

Case 80: He has tinnitus, and loves going to action movies. Some of the music and special effects are very loud. He looks at pre-molded and custom molded filtered earplugs. These types of plugs will screen out louder sound, and conversations will still be easy to hear. He decides on the pre-molded earplugs since they are lower cost, and feel comfortable in his ears.

Case 81: She has tinnitus and mild sound sensitivity. She feels better physically and mentally when she takes exercise classes at a local fitness studio. She finds the music played during classes is quite loud. She wants something comfortable that will let her hear the instructor's voice easily and not block out voices when she has conversations with friends in the class. She decides custom molded filtered earplugs are the best option for her.

Case 82: He has hearing loss and tinnitus. He loves going hunting for deer and moose. He always uses hearing protection when at the firing range sighting his rifle or target shooting. But he has never worn hearing protection while out hunting since it's only a few shots a year. He also needs to hear if animals are nearby for his own safety (e.g. hear twigs crackling from a nearby bear). His audiologist has warned him that even a few shots a year can damage his hearing permanently. He decides to try electronic protection so he can hear soft sounds and voices around him in the woods, but the protection will kick in instantly when he fires his gun. He chooses a model designed for hunting with camouflage pattern and shaped to fit well beside a rifle or shotgun in firing position.

Case 83: She has tinnitus and sound sensitivity. She spends a lot of time working with small children. She often has to listen to crying, screaming or shouting. She was using foam earplugs, but they made it hard to hear voices and she noticed her tinnitus was worse afterwards. She gradually switched over to custom molded filtered earplugs. She liked how these plugs sounded natural, and screened out the noise when the children were loud.

Case 84: He noticed that his tinnitus was worse after driving his car, especially when he left the window down during long drives. He decided to get pre-molded filtered earplugs that he could keep in the glove compartment. He could still hear the radio, passengers, and surrounding traffic. He found using the pre-molded filtered earplugs helped reduce tinnitus aggravation after driving.

Case 85: She has normal hearing. Restaurant noise always seemed bothersome, and her tinnitus always seemed worse after dinners out. She did not want to wear earmuffs while dining out. She decided to try pre-molded or custom molded filtered earplugs. Either would be inconspicuous and help cut the sound level, while letting her hear voices clearly.

Case 86: He had tinnitus and sound sensitivity. He hated vacuuming since he found it too loud, and his tinnitus was always worse afterwards. He decided to try high sound reduction earmuffs or foam earplugs that he could put on before turning the vacuum on, and then take off easily when he finished vacuuming. He preferred the earmuffs for convenience and re-usability. He also got a pair of custom molded filtered earplugs to use when he was around loud sound during other activities he found overly loud (e.g. at the dentist during drilling).

Case 87: She noticed her tinnitus seemed aggravated after using her hair dryer. She had tried foam earplugs that worked fine. She could re-use them for a fairly long time since her ears and fingers were always clean to put them in after having a shower. But sometimes they didn't fit right on the first try so it took some time to get them inserted properly. She decided to try banded earplugs that she could wear hanging under her chin. She could put them in before turning the dryer on, and then take them off easily when she turned the dryer off. They didn't get in the way much while she was styling her hair, and they lowered the sound to a more comfortable volume. She liked the convenience and re-usability, but she didn't like the sound when she accidentally bumped them with the hairdryer. She ended up switching to custom molded filtered earplugs.

CARING FOR TINNITUS

If I should pass the tomb of Jonah, I would stop and sit for a while. For I was buried one time deep in the dark, and came out alive after all. Author unknown.

JUST LEARN TO LIVE WITH IT

People with tinnitus would like to find a cure. But like chronic pain or other chronic conditions, tinnitus is not currently curable in the traditional sense. Rather than searching for cures, the best approach is for people to care for their tinnitus over time. All too often people are told, "Just learn to live with your tinnitus" without any information on how to take care of it. Caring for tinnitus doesn't mean fixing it or making your life perfect. Care means building coping strategies into your daily activities and routines. Coping starts with acceptance. Then the three main steps towards living better with tinnitus include intensive care, ongoing care and flare-up care.

ACCEPTANCE

A large part of acceptance is not only accepting that tinnitus is a chronic condition (at least until a cure is found), but also accepting that grief is a natural reaction. As discussed in the chapter on How We Hear Tinnitus, people dealing with tinnitus often don't realize that many of their emotional reactions are related to grief at diagnosis. People are told they have a condition that is not expected to go away. Natural reactions include sadness, anger, fear, worry, anxiety, and depression. These emotional reactions are the same as those seen with grief.

This is not at all surprising. Grief happens with any loss people experience as they go through life. Tinnitus certainly can involve a sense of loss, particularly the loss of silence.

It is important not to forget that grief or depression is not necessarily a negative thing. In his book *Care of The Soul*, Thomas Moore describes the role of depression through the ages. All humans have a range of emotions from sad (depressed) to happy. In the past, depression, sadness or melancholy were identified with the Roman god Saturn. But Saturn was also associated with wisdom, experience, and reflection. In ancient times depression was not necessarily considered good or bad. It was more a state of being and not necessarily a problem that needed to be eliminated.

Moore describes how even up to Renaissance times, some gardens had areas dedicated to Saturn. These were usually shady isolated places where people could go to experience feelings of sadness or depression without being disturbed. Our modern society usually encourages socialization and community. But our natural human range of emotions means that people often still need places where they can be alone to reflect on how they are feeling. It is honest to have melancholy or sad feelings. This is particularly true when people are dealing with conditions that involve visits to doctors, specialists, or hospitals. We may not be caring for ourselves properly if we don't accept this.

When dealing with tinnitus, people often move through stages of grieving. This process can be broken down into three simple stages: disbelief, distress and caring. The disbelief stage often starts with the diagnosis of tinnitus and the information that it is not expected to go away. This stage often involves thinking "This can't be true" or "Why me?" This disbelief is a common reaction to unpleasant news. It may last one or two months.

In the distress stage, negative emotions and feelings (e.g. sadness, worry and anger) can be more intense and prolonged and can seem overwhelming. During this painful distressing stage, people often become very focused on their tinnitus, and this is where negative emotional reactions to it can build up and become strong. This stage usually lasts about four months. But the distress stage is more likely to be longer lasting when people don't get appropriate education and reassurance about their tinnitus. If people become very distressed by their tinnitus, this stage can also last longer until tinnitus is treated and cared for appropriately.

Some people might move through the distress stage faster if they would observe how animals handle distress, pain, fear or anxiety. Animals often release their emotions physically. For example, a deer distressed by an attacking wolf may "pronk" after escaping. Pronking is when the deer makes high graceful leaps that help discharge "flight or fight" chemicals and calm the deer's system. Perhaps people would cope better with the painful stage of tinnitus related grief if they would also release their emotions physically. Cry. Yell. Punch a pillow. Run and jump around. Accepting and releasing emotions could help people move forward in their journey towards better coping.

In the third caring stage, there will still be disbelief and moments of pain, sadness, worry or anger. But people will have more interest in what is going on around them and are able to start planning ahead. This is the stage where people can actively start using coping strategies and treatment recommendations so that tinnitus moves away from being a central focus in their life.

It is in this caring stage that people need to recognize that no matter what they do their tinnitus is going to fluctuate. Like other long term conditions (e.g. chronic pain), tinnitus will have ups and downs over time. These fluctuations have nothing to do with anything except for the tinnitus. Before treatment, tinnitus distress typically swings up and down with these fluctuations leading to little or no long-term change for the better. Reacting with grief to natural changes in tinnitus loudness will only prolong the distress. Reacting with appropriate coping strategies is the best way to learn to live with tinnitus. Figure 1 illustrates the natural ups and downs of tinnitus distress for a person who is not caring for their tinnitus and who is not coping well with their severe tinnitus most of the time.

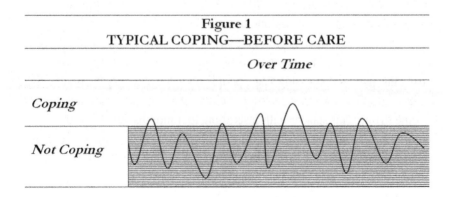

Figure 1
TYPICAL COPING—BEFORE CARE

Over Time

Coping

Not Coping

Difficulty coping and tinnitus distress can be compared to difficulty coping and stress. Some speakers on stress management use the example of holding up a small glass full of water and asking people to guess how much it weighs. But the point is that the weight doesn't matter. What matters is how long you try to hold up the glass. If you hold it for a minute, that's not a problem. If you hold it for an hour, you'll have an ache in your arm. If you hold it for a day, you'll have to call an ambulance. In each case it's the same weight, but the longer you hold it, the heavier the burden becomes. It's the same for stress management. If we carry our burdens all the time, sooner or later, as the burden becomes increasingly heavy then we won't be able to carry on. With tinnitus, it doesn't matter how loud the tinnitus is or how it sounds. Distress happens because people have trouble letting go of negative emotional reactions to their tinnitus. They carry the burden of listening and reacting to their tinnitus until distress can become severe.

Obviously, the best solution for people not coping with their tinnitus is to learn strategies to help them cope better. Carrying the burden of tinnitus distress without purpose is torture, but tinnitus care with purpose is a gateway to progress. Research shows that when people with tinnitus learn effective coping strategies they show significant improvement in well-being. Strategy is sometimes defined in dictionaries as a plan for reaching a goal. Strategy is also defined as military methods used to meet enemies under conditions beneficial to your own forces. Tinnitus treatment gives you an individual plan to reach your end goal of better coping. By using a treatment plan, you also create conditions beneficial to yourself to help overcome any tinnitus distress. It is all a matter of caring for your tinnitus as you live your daily life. The first plan of attack is intensive care.

INTENSIVE CARE

As discussed in earlier chapters, tinnitus treatment approaches may include education and reassurance, hearing loss management, sound enrichment, mind enrichment, body enrichment, sleep management and hearing protection management. These approaches may be used alone or in combination. People may need one appointment or multiple appointments. The more severe the tinnitus distress, the more likely multiple treatment approaches and multiple appointments will be needed. The end goal of any treatment is reduced tinnitus distress and better coping. Initially with treatment a person's emotional reaction to their tinnitus (e.g. worry, fear, anxiety, depression, anger, etc.) should gradually reduce. People get used to their tinnitus so they are no longer annoyed or distressed by it even though the tinnitus may have the same loudness and pitch as before treatment. After the emotional reaction changes, the percentage of time when you are aware of tinnitus typically decreases significantly.

When people with tinnitus start treatment, an intense comprehensive approach is usually taken. They might start to use hearing aids. They might use sound enrichment day and night. They might use mind enrichment or body enrichment strategies. They might go to regular treatment or counselling sessions. They may start using strategies in their daily life to help relax and to help distract themselves from their tinnitus. They may change their sleep routine. They may change the type of hearing protection they have been using. In some cases, they might also use prescription drugs to help get them started coping better.

As discussed in previous chapters, prescription drugs can be used to reduce emotional reactions to tinnitus. There are medications available that can be used to help with any anxiety, depression and poor sleep that can contribute to distress. If used appropriately under medical guidance, prescription drugs can be helpful for initial intensive care. The goal is to eventually phase out the use of these drugs after other strategies are built into the overall treatment plan. Again, phasing out use of prescription drugs should only be done under medical guidance.

It is important to remember that starting treatment (self-help or formal) will not mean instant improvement in tinnitus. Some people do notice improvement fairly quickly. But it is also common for tinnitus to seem worse with initial treatment. One might make an analogy to pain in these cases. For example, if you have injured yourself, you might be in severe pain. If you had physiotherapy, you might also feel pain after appointments as your therapist gives you treatment or exercises to complete. But the pain is often different. People often describe it as a "good pain" as healing starts to take place. Don't feel discouraged if your tinnitus seems louder after you start using coping strategies, hearing aids, or devices. This is a positive sign that your auditory system is responding by reacting differently.

It can be exhausting to go through this initial intensive care. Change is always difficult, particularly when results are not instant. If you are going through formal therapy, it is essential to attend treatment at recommended intervals. Otherwise it is easy to forget information covered during counselling. If you have been fit with devices (e.g. hearing aids, tabletop sound machine, in-ear sound generators or combination instruments), follow-up visits are important to have devices adjusted as needed over time as well as to make sure you are using devices properly. Some of the counselling may be done by telephone if people live a distance from their care provider.

It can be misleading in early stages of intensive tinnitus care or treatment to rely on "spot checks" of tinnitus status to monitor progress. While spot checks of distress rankings are routinely used to monitor treatment progress, they must be interpreted correctly. I have seen cases where people have sunk into a deep depression when ranking scales used to evaluate their tinnitus distress seemed to show initial improvement and then later "worsening" after months of treatment. This apparent worsening is certainly not an indication that treatment has been useless. It is essential to keep the big picture in mind and look at long-term trends instead of a few snapshots over time.

> ***Example—Changes with Intensive Care***: This man had severe tinnitus distress. He was referred for formal tinnitus treatment (sound therapy and counselling therapy). At his initial appointment he had a 90% tinnitus distress ranking (high distress). At his 3 month appointment, he had a 64% distress ranking (less distress). But then at his 6 month appointment, he had an 80% distress ranking. If wrongly interpreted, his 6 month appointment appears to show a relapse despite treatment. Correctly interpreted, treatment is working:

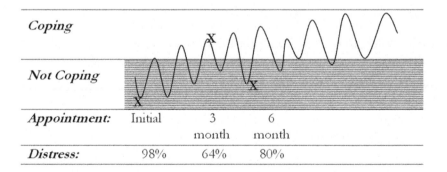

Appointment:	Initial	3 month	6 month
Distress:	98%	64%	80%

The fact that the 3 month appointment showed significant improvement is a very positive indicator that this person's tinnitus was responding to treatment. His 6 month appointment results were just a snapshot taken at a different point in his tinnitus distress cycle. Tinnitus follows natural ups and downs and flare-ups happen. Ongoing care in the long-term would lead to a return to lower distress.

Author's Case: After months of intensive care, I tried not to pay attention or listen to my tinnitus. Then one day when I checked on it, I noticed a big change in the volume and pitch. Suddenly the tinnitus was no longer screeching at me. I went from not coping towards coping. But instead of feeling happy, I was surprised to feel an unexpected sense of loss. I don't know if this is common, because I have never seen any mention of this by anybody else with tinnitus. I kept checking to see if my tinnitus had completely disappeared. It was still there, and within days had accelerated right back up to it's original screeching. Once again I was not coping. I felt frustrated, disappointed and angry that after months of coping strategies, there didn't appear to be any benefit. Then I took a deep breath, and went back to following my intensive care plan. Within a month, the tinnitus decreased back down again. It is always there when I check on it. But after months and years of using my treatment toolbox, I am rarely distressed by tinnitus anymore.

ONGOING CARE

Over time intensive care leads into ongoing care. Certain components of intensive care may not be necessary continuously. For example, people won't need to keep taking daily prescription drugs to help them sleep. They won't need regular counselling sessions or appointments with their tinnitus care provider. Some people are able to change how they are using devices. They might switch from combination instruments to regular hearing aids plus environmental sound enrichment. Sometimes people gradually stop using coping strategies because they are managing better. For example, they might forget to use sound enrichment continuously throughout their day since they are not noticing their tinnitus much. They may stop regularly using distraction or relaxation techniques.

This change in care intensity over time is similar to caring for chronic pain or other chronic conditions. For example, a person with severe chronic pain may begin with an intensive care program of strong prescription painkillers, physiotherapy, braces, canes, specific rehabilitation exercises, etc. With ongoing care, they may use different or weaker prescription painkillers, over the counter painkillers, braces only for difficult activities (e.g. long walks, gardening), less intensive maintenance exercises, etc. Figure 2 illustrates the natural ups and downs of tinnitus for a person moving from intensive to ongoing care.

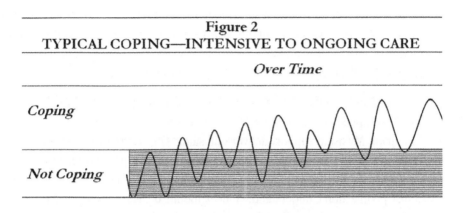

Figure 2
TYPICAL COPING—INTENSIVE TO ONGOING CARE

Over Time

Coping

Not Coping

Even with ongoing care, tinnitus distress will still swing up and down regardless of tinnitus intensity. It is the nature of the beast. But over time, the downs are not as bad and will not last as long when coping strategies and devices are used. More time is spent coping well and less time is spent not coping. Coping and general well-being will significantly improve overall with ongoing tinnitus care.

FLARE-UP CARE

With treatment life does not become problem free. But over time, treatment should help with problem solving. Even with effective intensive and ongoing care, there will still be times when a person's tinnitus distress increases and they have trouble coping. These are often referred to as "flare-ups". Flare-ups could be from natural increases in the tinnitus fluctuation cycle or be from various triggers. Triggers can include change in hearing, change in health (e.g. from minor cold to major disease), death in family, change in work situation, financial worries, etc. These triggers often increase stress and this can increase difficulty coping.

This increased coping difficulty can lead to distress and a return to grieving. Flare-ups may cause people to re-experience the sadness or other emotions that they went through when they were diagnosed or when they found out their tinnitus was not curable. This renewed grief can come from the need for further intensive care during flare-ups. People often feel relief and satisfaction at their coping ability when they move past intensive care into ongoing care. The thought of returning to more intensive care when a flare-up happens (e.g. more appointments, more use of devices, more counselling, more strategies) can cause various reactions including depression, sadness and exhaustion as well as frustration. But this is all part of the journey. Learning how to handle flare-ups will only improve your ongoing care over time.

> **Author's Case:** Even after years of using coping strategies, I still get flare-ups sometimes. Recently, I had a severe increase in tinnitus and pain. My usual support network all said, "Oh, you're just stressed out". Knowing that stress is a trigger does not make the tinnitus any less or make the flare-up go away. It only makes me feel all alone that most people don't understand. After a month of using my intensive care strategies with no effect, I was depressed and frustrated. I went to see my family doctor. A prescription medication was recommended for sleep. I also started using some techniques that I hadn't tried before. These included a cognitive technique to stop negative "What if" thinking, a different distraction technique I hadn't tried before, and a different relaxation technique at bedtime. Gradually over time, this combination of strategies helped settle down the flare-up. The most useful strategies will be added into my toolbox as "everyday tools". Other strategies will stay in my toolbox until I need them again as "flare-up tools".

When flare-ups happen, they won't last as long or be as distressing if you continue to use effective strategies to care for your tinnitus. Records of which treatments have been tried and how well they worked can definitely come in handy. What worked initially for intensive care? Are you still using it? Can you use it again during flare-ups? If necessary, it is often very helpful to return to your audiologist, tinnitus specialist, and/or counselling specialist. These care providers can help you work through flare-ups. Some providers call these "booster visits" since they can help boost you over a rough patch. Many people also have supportive family or friends they can reach out to during a flare-up.

Part of tinnitus care is making adjustments to your tinnitus treatment plan over time. When tinnitus care is successful, the person will be able to cope even during the natural ups and downs of daily life. As Louisa May Alcott once said, "I'm not afraid of storms, for I'm learning how to sail my ship". Figure 3 illustrates the natural ups and downs of tinnitus for a person successfully caring for their tinnitus even through flare-ups.

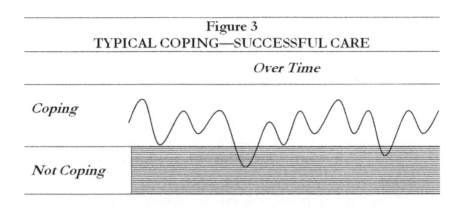

Figure 3
TYPICAL COPING—SUCCESSFUL CARE

Over Time

Coping

Not Coping

As discussed earlier in this chapter, in his book *Care of the Soul* Thomas Moore describes how the Roman god Saturn was associated with some negative emotions. Moore goes on to describe how these emotions can still be used towards change. Carpenters building new foundations and structures were often associated with Saturn. Moving away from distress may mean new foundations and structures in your life as you build up coping strategies and techniques. Take care of yourself and your tinnitus. Follow any recommended medical or dental treatment. Aid your hearing if necessary. Enrich or keep your ears busy with better sound. Enrich or keep your mind busy with better thoughts. Take care of your body. Protect your ears from hazardous noise. Live your life. If your tinnitus increases with stress, then let your tinnitus guide you in when you need to take better care of yourself in all areas of your life. Use every tool at your disposal to live without distress and cope well. Keep in mind the words of the 18th century English author Samuel Johnson: "Great works are performed, not by strength, but by perseverance."

Author's Case: Day and night tinnitus distress.

Intensive Care: All day sound enrichment (e.g. music, TV); all day mind enrichment (e.g. distraction techniques whenever thoughts of tinnitus entered my mind); relaxation techniques (e.g. before falling asleep at night); all night sound enrichment (white noise); sleep management techniques; body enrichment techniques (e.g. exercise); appropriate hearing protection when in hazardous noise.

Ongoing Care: Daytime sound enrichment as needed; all night sound enrichment (white noise); body enrichment techniques (e.g. exercise); hearing protection when in hazardous noise.

Flare-up Care: Similar to intensive care.

Case 88: Hearing loss, day and night tinnitus distress, and sound sensitivity.

Intensive Care: Medication to help with anxiety and sleep; formal counselling sessions with Tinnitus Retraining Therapy specialist; ear level combination instruments (hearing aids plus white noise) and environmental sound enrichment for day; hearing aids eventually phased in for day instead of the combination instruments; white noise bedside tabletop sound machine for night.

Ongoing Care: Hearing aids and environmental sound enrichment for day; white noise bedside tabletop sound machine for night.

Flare-up Care: Combination instruments instead of hearing aids until flare-up settles down; medication for anxiety or sleep as needed; additional counselling sessions as needed.

Case 89: Hearing loss and is bothered by tinnitus sometimes during his day.

Intensive Care: Education and reassurance from audiologist; hearing aids; environmental sound enrichment; distraction techniques.

Ongoing Care: Hearing aids.

Flare-up Care: Additional environmental sound enrichment and distraction techniques; additional counselling as needed.

Case 90: Day and night tinnitus distress.

Intensive Care: Counselling from tinnitus music therapy provider (e.g. Neuromonics Tinnitus Treatment); music based device for day and night.

Ongoing Care: Environmental sound enrichment and healthy lifestyle.

Flare-up Care: Additional use of music-based device until flare-up settles down; additional counselling sessions as needed.

Case 91: Severe sound sensitivity.

Intensive Care: Formal counselling sessions (Cognitive Behaviour Therapy) with psychologist; pink noise through audio equipment for day; pink noise sound machine for night; phase out constant use of foam earplugs, and phase in use of filtered earplugs for loud environments; relaxation techniques.

Ongoing Care: Pink noise sound machine for night; filtered earplugs for loud daytime environments; relaxation techniques.

Flare-up Care: Additional use of pink noise for day until flare-up settles down; additional counselling sessions as needed.

Case 92: Hearing loss and tinnitus that is bothersome sometimes during the day.

Intensive Care: Counselling on tinnitus from audiologist; hearing aids; environmental sound enrichment; electronic earmuffs for work instead of traditional earmuffs; reduce caffeine intake from 12 cups of coffee per day to as low as possible.

Ongoing Care: Hearing aids; appropriate hearing protection; maintain healthy lifestyle.

Flare-up Care: Additional environmental sound enrichment and counselling as needed.

Case 93: Hearing loss and tinnitus that is bothersome during the day and when trying to sleep.

Intensive Care: Education and reassurance on tinnitus from audiologist; hearing aids; environmental sound enrichment for day; white noise bedside tabletop sound machine for night; formal Cognitive Behavioural Therapy from psychologist.

Ongoing Care: Hearing aids; environmental sound enrichment; white noise bedside tabletop sound machine.

Flare-up Care: Additional use of Cognitive Behavioural Therapy techniques; additional counselling as needed.

Case 94: Tinnitus for years, and is used to it.

Intensive Care: None required.

Ongoing Care: Carry on with his daily life.

Flare-up Care: Ignore it and carry on with daily life.

Case 95: Tinnitus that is distressing sometimes when trying to fall asleep.

Intensive Care: Education and reassurance on tinnitus from audiologist; relaxation sound enrichment for night.

Ongoing Care: Carry on with usual lifestyle.

Flare-up Care: Use relaxation sound enrichment as needed.

Case 96: Hearing loss and tinnitus distress in general.

Intensive Care: Progressive Tinnitus Management counselling and guidance from audiologist; hearing aids; environmental sound enrichment for day; sound machine for night.

Ongoing Care: Hearing aids.

Flare-up Care: Environmental sound enrichment for day and sound machine for night; additional counselling as needed. This person was advised that if they used the sound machine on a regular nightly basis for ongoing care, they would likely reduce the number of flare-ups over time.

Case 97: Worried about tinnitus.

Intensive Care: Counselling on tinnitus; environmental sound enrichment, mind enrichment (e.g. hobbies and activities).

Ongoing Care: Healthy lifestyle and enjoyment of hobbies.

Flare-up Care: Additional environmental sound enrichment; additional counselling as needed.

SELECTING A CARE PROVIDER

If one is truly to succeed in leading a person to a specific place, one must first and foremost take care to find him where he is and begin there. Søren Kierkegaard.

Many people with tinnitus or sound sensitivity are able to use a self-help approach once they know what tools and strategies are available and appropriate to use. To help them reach the point of self-managing, the guidance of a care provider is helpful. As discussed in the chapter on Tinnitus Evaluation, treatment planning will depend on evaluation findings and your specific concerns. Your family doctor and ear specialist should rule out any medical issues before starting any treatment. Your dentist may also be involved if dental issues are present. Once the focus is on non-medical treatment, there is usually one primary tinnitus care provider involved, similar to how your family doctor is your primary medical care provider.

Audiologists are most commonly the primary care provider for people with tinnitus or sound sensitivity. Some audiologists are tinnitus specialists who offer a single therapy approach or philosophy (e.g. Tinnitus Retraining Therapy, Tinnitus Music Therapy, etc.). Formal specialized treatment is usually offered through a tinnitus clinic. But there are typically a limited number of formally trained tinnitus specialists working in tinnitus clinics. Usually these clinics are found in large urban cities. Formal therapy is highly recommended for people with severe distress or complex issues. But many people can't attend specialized formal therapy for various reasons including lack of tinnitus clinics in their local geographical area or financial cost (e.g. treatment and travel related).

Other audiologists use basic principles of different treatment approaches. Audiologists often work in various local hearing clinics or hospitals. Even if they don't have formal specialized training, these professionals can be great resources. Audiologists can counsel their clients on tinnitus, hearing loss and communication strategies. They can help educate their clients on available treatment, and recommend and provide appropriate treatment tools. They can guide their clients on how best to use various devices and strategies. They can make referrals to other professionals as needed. Often the audiologist works as part of a team including ear specialists (e.g. Otologist or Otolaryngologist) and counselling specialists (e.g. psychologists, psychiatrists).

Experts suggest that the success of treatment depends in large part on the relationship with the care provider. You should feel comfortable and supported by your tinnitus or sound sensitivity care provider just as you would by your doctor or any other health professional you are dealing with on a long-term basis (e.g. chiropractor, massage therapist, etc.). Because the relationship with your care provider is so important, there are several factors to consider when choosing your audiologist or primary care provider. These factors include experience, kindness, time, and hope.

EXPERIENCE

There is no substitute for a care provider who is knowledgeable about tinnitus or sound sensitivity treatment approaches and has experience with them. An audiologist or tinnitus specialist who understands the principles behind currently available treatment methods can best adapt tinnitus or sound sensitivity management approaches for each individual person. Experienced care providers can explain pros and cons of various treatments or approaches. By being informed, people can then work together with their care provider to make educated decisions about what their own treatment plan should include. Individualized treatment plans are most successful in reducing distress.

KINDNESS

People often don't consider kindness when selecting a care provider. But some providers are uncomfortable with discussing feelings or distress, and may be inclined to give pep talks (e.g. it's not that bad, it could be worse, etc.) rather than truly listening with kindness. A kind provider is often empathetic.

Empathy is when a person is able to relate to your feelings or situation. Tinnitus specialists in general are very kind and empathetic towards people with tinnitus or sound sensitivity. It is helpful to find an audiologist or care provider who is an empathetic and kind person.

TIME

As discussed in the chapter on Caring for Tinnitus, treatment takes time. Formal treatment may take 6 months to 2 years to complete, and ongoing "booster" visits may still be needed when flare-ups happen. Tinnitus specialists may spend at least 2 hours (particularly initially) in evaluating your tinnitus or sound sensitivity and in providing education and reassurance. Follow-up appointments are often at least 30 to 60 minutes long depending on the issues or concerns that need to be addressed. Some providers encourage clients to contact them by phone or e-mail so they can respond quickly to concerns as they come up.

At a local audiology clinic, your appointments with your audiologist would typically be at least 15 to 30 minutes long depending on what is being addressed at the appointment. If your hearing aid needs adjustments but you also want to discuss your tinnitus or sound sensitivity, it helps if you make the clinic aware so that they can schedule time for that conversation. Choose an audiologist who gives you the time to talk about concerns whether you are starting out with a treatment plan or working through a flare-up.

There is nothing worse than going to a provider, and walking out of an appointment feeling as if the person didn't spend sufficient time with you, your questions were left unanswered, or the person didn't seem that interested in discussing or addressing your concerns. This is where the experience, kindness and time come in. Tinnitus is a long-term condition, and sound sensitivity takes time to treat. You need to choose a care provider you can be comfortable with over the long-term. You will likely be spending a lot of time with them.

HOPE

Research shows that people get the best results from treatment when they feel hopeful about the outcome. This hope helps them adjust as they use coping strategies and techniques. People can take control and influence how they are managing their tinnitus or sound sensitivity. It is easier to move forward with treatment if you feel hopeful about the future.

J. L. Mayes

SUMMARY

An individualized treatment plan gives people the tools they need (strategies and devices) to cope better. Some believe that tinnitus treatment should never be provided outside a tinnitus clinic or by anyone except a formally trained tinnitus specialist. This is not always an option for people due to cost, travel, or other individual reasons. It is proven that audiologists and other care providers (e.g. counselling specialists) can help people with tinnitus cope better even if those professionals don't have specific specialized tinnitus treatment training. When choosing an audiologist or tinnitus specialist you may want to consider the following:

- Is the provider knowledgeable about current tinnitus or sound sensitivity treatment options including cost and availability?
- Do they have knowledge or experience on how to fit hearing aids or devices for people with tinnitus (or sound sensitivity)?
- Are they able to put together an individualized treatment plan?
- Does the provider have a positive attitude that treatment is beneficial?
- Are they open to discussing promising new therapies?
- Does the provider have tinnitus or have they coped with a chronic condition?
- Can they spend time with you over the long term?
- Are they willing to work together with you to problem solve your issues?
- Are appointments long enough?
- Does the provider explain results and findings?
- Are your questions answered, or if time is short, does the provider arrange another time to discuss your concerns?
- Is telephone counselling available if necessary (e.g. to reduce travel)?
- Is the care provider a good listener?
- Do you feel comfortable sharing concerns?
- Is the care provider kind and empathetic?
- Do they help you feel hopeful?

It is important to remember that the care provider is there to guide you, but that you should not give your tinnitus over to them just because they are an "authority". As Albert Einstein once said, "All knowledge of reality starts from experience and ends in it". You know yourself and what you are experiencing better than anybody else. So you need to be actively involved in planning and participating in the treatment process, and continue to use your tinnitus (or sound sensitivity) tools and coping strategies over time even after formal treatment ends.

Since treatment is based on each person's own experience of tinnitus or sound sensitivity, I often think it is best to have a treatment "coach". A coach is someone who can train and motivate you to achieve your personal best. The relationship with your care provider is essential to help you reach your best coping ability possible. Your care provider can help you choose the tools that speak directly to your needs for your individual treatment toolbox. Select a care provider who is experienced, kind and who spends time with you to problem-solve. This can bring hope and a better quality of life into your journey as you care for your tinnitus or sound sensitivity.

Author's Case: I was once referred to a specialist. As I waited in the examining room, I noticed I was sitting beside a dirty old pot full of what appeared to be an ancient stew. The physician spent so little time with me that I did not feel he had a good understanding of my concerns. He did not come across as kind or empathetic. Although he recommended treatment, I was not at all hopeful that it would help since I had no faith in him and I never wanted to see him again.

A different care provider took time to listen and understand my concerns. He then asked me if I was "appointmented out" since I was in the process of having multiple appointments with different professionals for tests, therapy and follow-up. I was in fact exhausted of appointments. He helped me decide which appointments and devices were essential and which could wait. His empathy and kindness certainly gave me hope, and helped me cope better.

Other Cases: The author has clients who have seen various care providers for their tinnitus or sound sensitivity. Most prefer getting treatment from an audiologist, tinnitus specialist or counselling specialist who is knowledgeable and kind, who spends time with them, and who gives them hope for improved coping and well-being in the future.

ALTERNATIVE APPROACHES

The human race has one really effective weapon, and that is laughter. Mark Twain.

Hearing loss management, sound enrichment, mind enrichment, body enrichment, sleep management and hearing protection management are all scientifically proven methods of tinnitus care. They improve coping over the long term. People with tinnitus or sound sensitivity are often interested in other remedies or treatments that may advertise a cure or rapid relief. They may focus on these apparent "quick fixes" instead of using proven coping strategies and treatment approaches. Do not seek treatment from anybody offering false promises or claims of a cure, since there is no cure at the current time. See the chapter on Future Hope for information on promising research that may one day lead to a cure.

Some people have an interest in alternative or complementary therapy approaches to help them cope better. Usually reported benefit for many approaches is based on anecdotal or personal reports rather than well-controlled scientific studies. People who think they were helped are quick to speak up, while people who weren't helped tend not to say anything. So in general, personal reports don't help much in figuring out what might benefit other individuals. When scientific studies on alternative approaches are available, the difficulty is that data is analyzed based on the entire group of people studied. Often no overall group benefit may be found even though certain individuals within the group may have shown some improvement with a particular therapy.

With any approach, people can also experience the Hawthorne Effect. This effect is when people experience a sense of relief or improvement just because someone is doing something for them. As discussed in the chapter on Selecting a Care Provider, the time, kindness, and hope offered by any provider might help a person feel better about their tinnitus regardless of the treatment itself.

The following information is provided to help you make more informed decisions if you are considering alternative tinnitus care approaches. Some approaches may also be helpful for people with sound sensitivity, particularly those that help with relaxation, stress reduction or improving feelings of well-being. If you are planning to explore an alternative approach, you should discuss it with your audiologist or tinnitus specialist. You should also get medical clearance from your family doctor or ear specialist. Any doctors or care providers you see for any reason must always be informed about any alternative remedies you are using. Alternative approaches may not be allowed at the same time as some formal treatment programs. Be cautious about using alternative approaches instead of other proven treatment methods. If you do decide to try an alternative approach, research it first (e.g. cost, side effects, etc.) and make sure the person treating you is qualified and reputable.

Acupuncture and **Acupressure** are two commonly used alternative approaches. Acupuncture is an ancient Chinese healing system that uses fine needles inserted into the body at specific therapy points. Acupressure is a healing system similar to acupuncture. It uses gentle pressure on specific pressure points on the body instead of needles.

In Mark Evans book *The Guide to Natural Therapies*, he includes photographs illustrating an acupressure point for tinnitus. It is just in front of the outer ear at the middle point. This point is near the hinge of the jaw. If you are touching the right spot you will be able to feel your bottom jaw moving just below your finger when you open and close your mouth. Based on the author's experience, people with tinnitus often have a hard spot there like a very small grain of sugar or frozen pea. The hardness disappears with very gentle touch or pressure. Various books or courses on acupressure also illustrate therapy points for the ear or tinnitus.

Whether therapy points help with tinnitus or not, acupuncture or acupressure treatment in general can improve relaxation and that can improve coping.

Alexander Technique was developed by an actor named Frederick Alexander. It is a method of training how we use our bodies (posture, body movement, positioning) to improve how our internal organs function as well as improve overall health. This technique might help with well-being in general.

Amalgam (Mercury) Dental Fillings are "silver" or metal fillings that contain a high percentage of mercury. There is some controversy over their safety. These dental fillings may contribute to various chronic health problems. Research suggests that mercury vapour from these fillings can affect the hearing system over the long term. Some people with tinnitus report lower tinnitus severity after having their amalgam fillings replaced with fillings that do not contain mercury. There can be complications or side effects from having mercury fillings removed. Dentists experienced in this procedure can discuss risks, safety precautions, and often provide recommendations on how to detoxify your body afterwards if you have the removal done. People with tinnitus or sound sensitivity may want to avoid getting amalgam fillings in the first place if possible.

Antioxidants are substances that help protect the cells in our bodies from damage. Antioxidants help maintain health and prevent disease. Some research suggests that antioxidants may be effective in protecting the ears from noise related hearing damage. Food sources of antioxidants mainly include fruits and vegetables including green leafy, orange and red coloured (e.g. carrots, sweet potatoes, mangos, tomatoes, spinach, kale, etc.). Other foods (e.g. certain meats, fish, breads, grains, nuts, dairy products, oils, etc.) may also contain antioxidants. A diet that includes recommended daily amounts of antioxidants is likely helpful for overall health including ear health.

Retail products containing antioxidants are available, and may be marketed as a "hearing protection" pill. While this type of product may help protect the hearing by strengthening the ears natural defenses, anyone exposed to hazardous noise should always use appropriate hearing protection. (See chapter on Hearing Protection Management.) Any antioxidant vitamins or supplements should not be taken without clearance from a medical doctor.

Aromatherapy is an ancient approach used to heal and balance people's body systems. In ancient times aromatic plants were burned to "smoke" illness out, and aromatic plants and extracts have been used by various ancient civilizations. This approach might help with well-being in general.

Auditory Nerve Surgery involves cutting or destroying the auditory or hearing nerve. It is not an appropriate tinnitus treatment. This type of surgery is sometimes necessary for reasons that have nothing to do with having tinnitus. It makes a person completely deaf in the ear with the cut nerve. It has also been found that cutting the auditory nerve causes tinnitus in over half of people who did not have tinnitus before the operation.

B Vitamin levels may be low in some people with tinnitus. Research has not found any beneficial effect in general when people with tinnitus take B Vitamin supplements, although certain individuals might have some benefit. Some research suggests these vitamins might help the ears be better protected from noise damage. People may want to consider taking a regular daily vitamin and mineral supplement that contains B vitamins to maintain healthy levels in your system. It is not recommended that people with tinnitus take "mega-doses" of any supplement. Any vitamins or supplements should not be taken without clearance from a medical doctor.

Biofeedback or mind-body therapy trains people to use their mind to control various body functions including brain activity, blood pressure, muscle tension, heart rate, etc. It is particularly useful in treating stress-related conditions. Since tinnitus and sound sensitivity are aggravated by stress, this approach could be helpful for some people. By gaining control over their body, people often also feel more in control of their life in general. Even with practice, certain people are better at using biofeedback techniques than others. Some experts suggest that biofeedback is not helpful when used alone, but is useful in combination with other coping strategies.

Black Cohosh is an herbal remedy most often used to treat menopausal symptoms and arthritis. People with tinnitus sometimes use it. Research has not found any beneficial effect in general. Any drugs (include herbal treatments) should not be taken without clearance and supervision from a medical doctor.

Chiropractic involves manual adjustment techniques (usually along the spine) to treat musculoskeletal pain (e.g. back pain, neck pain, headaches, migraines, etc.). Some people report that chiropractic helps their tinnitus. In people with tinnitus and musculoskeletal pain, chiropractic could help with coping in general since pain reduction can lead to better well-being overall.

Cochlear Implants are devices surgically implanted in the inner ear. The devices improve sound perception and speech understanding in people with severe to profound hearing loss that can't be helped by traditional hearing aids. Cochlear implants are not intended to be a tinnitus treatment, although these implants can reduce tinnitus in many people once the implant is activated after surgery. Some people have tinnitus start after the surgery, and sometimes the surgery makes tinnitus worse. People with cochlear implants and distressing tinnitus can develop an individual tinnitus treatment plan based on their individual needs.

Cranio-Sacral Therapy involves gentle manipulations of the skull to treat various conditions including headaches, migraines, jaw pain, and recurrent ear or sinus infections in children. It may be available through osteopaths or chiropractors. This approach might help with pain relief and health in general for people with tinnitus and head pain.

Creative Visualization is a method of using mental images or pictures to help improve various areas of a person's life including their health. It is often used as a specific method to increase positive thinking. Creative visualization can help some people feel more in control and have a more positive outlook on life, and that can improve coping.

Cued Speech is a hand positioning system that helps make the sounds of speech more visible for people with hearing loss or with problems hearing in difficult listening situations. The system includes eight hand shapes that can be used in four different positions. The person talking uses the hand shapes near their face or mouth. This helps the listener see the difference between speech sounds (especially consonants) that are hard to hear. For example, if a listener thought the speaker said, "pat" when they actually said "cat", the speaker could use the hand shape for "c" while speaking to make it easier to distinguish. The listener and their most frequent conversational partners would need to learn the system and practice using it regularly to become good at it.

Cued speech has been adapted for approximately 60 languages and dialects. Cued speech is mainly used by people who communicate through speech and hearing. It is not a full sign language like those used by people in the deaf community who mainly communicate through signing. As an alternative to cued speech, some people learn and use sign language alphabets so they can spell out a word that is misheard or hard to hear. Cued speech or simple alphabet signs can help make conversation easier and improve communication, which can lower stress and improve coping. Various books and Websites have information on Cued Speech or sign language alphabets.

Ear Candling or **Ear Coning** is an alternate approach that is said to remove earwax. Earwax naturally moves out the ear canal on its own along with any dirt or other matter. Ear candling uses a special cone shaped candle placed in the ear canal while a person is lying down. The burning wick and smoke supposedly extracts earwax and impurities from the ear. Some people even say that impurities are withdrawn from the head and sinus cavities while candling, although this is physically (anatomically) impossible. Experiments have shown that all "residue" comes from the candle itself. Risks include burns, wax blockages in the ear canal, and holes in the eardrum. Ear candling or ear coning is NEVER recommended for anyone. Excess earwax should only be removed by a qualified and trained professional using appropriate methods. Discuss any concerns about excess earwax with your family doctor or audiologist. In some cases, a referral to an ear specialist may be needed.

Food Allergies have been linked with tinnitus. Food can cause various reactions in the body including headaches, stomach problems, respiratory problems, etc. Allergic reactions may appear immediately (e.g. hives, anaphylactic shock, etc.) or may cause a more chronic reaction (e.g. headaches, arthritis, asthma, fatigue, depression, etc.). People may also have food intolerances when they react negatively to a certain food (e.g. stomach problems from lactose intolerance, migraines from red wine, etc.). If you suspect you have food allergies or intolerances, you should see a qualified professional (e.g. allergy specialist). Treatment for food allergies can improve overall health and may also reduce tinnitus in some cases.

Fractal Music is a special type of pleasant relaxing music. The music is manipulated by an algorithm or mathematical equation so that the music repeats in an irregular or unpredictable way. The musical notes repeat enough to sound familiar but vary enough not to sound repetitive. There are no sudden changes in tone or tempo. Most people find fractal music soothing or relaxing. Although research evidence is not yet available, fractal music could likely be a beneficial relaxation sound type to use for sound enrichment. Certain hearing aid manufacturers are now including relaxing fractal music as a program option on their hearing aids (although these hearing aids are not currently being specifically marketed as a tinnitus treatment).

Gingko Biloba is the most popular herbal treatment for tinnitus. In Europe the use of gingko biloba for people with tinnitus is widespread. Europeans typically use gingko biloba along with other treatment approaches. Large scale research studies on this herb have found no beneficial effect in general although certain individuals do report reduced tinnitus after taking gingko biloba. Many available studies used different dosages or had flaws in how the study was carried out, which makes it hard to prove any benefit of this herb. Gingko biloba could interact with other prescription medications, and can have side effects including indigestion, depression and potential cardiovascular or heart related effects. Any drugs (include this type of herbal treatment) should never be taken without clearance and supervision from a medical doctor.

Homeopathy was developed back in the 1700's by Dr. Edward Bach. It is a form of treatment that uses various gentle flower or plant-based remedies to promote self-healing. Although research has failed to come up with an explanation for the effectiveness of Bach remedies, it is accepted that there is a physiological basis for its benefits. This approach might help with health and well-being in general.

Hypnosis or **Hypnotherapy** probably dates back to the 1700's, and involves concentrating the mind to create a state of deep relaxation. Hypnotherapy is primarily used for stress reduction and improved relaxation. It seems to work better for some people than for others. Hypnosis or hypnotherapy may help some people cope better. Relaxation techniques like hypnotherapy are believed to be most effective when used in combination with other techniques rather than being used alone.

Inversion Therapy or "upside down" therapy uses the force of gravity to stretch the body and increase blood flow to the upper extremities (e.g. brain). This type of therapy often uses an inversion table that a person lies on and then tilts so that they are in an inverted position with their feet higher than their head. At the greatest extent, a person can invert or tilt completely upside down. It is not necessary to be completely upside down for inversion therapy. A therapeutic effect is possible as long as you are lying with your body on a slant with your feet higher than your head. Some people use a slant board. This is a sturdy board with one end placed on the ground and the other end placed safely and securely on an elevated surface (e.g. on the first step of a staircase, on a bed, etc.). People could get in a similar position by lying on a hill with their head downhill and their feet uphill.

Inversion therapy increases oxygen and blood flow to the brain and hearing system. This may make tinnitus seem louder while a person is inverted or tilted. It stimulates all regions of the inner ear balance system including the upper regions that may not get much stimulation from other everyday positions (e.g. standing, sitting, walking, lying down). Inversion therapy is reported to have various benefits from reducing back pain, headaches, stress and depression to better circulation, mental alertness and balance. People who use inversion therapy often report that it gives them improved physical and mental well-being. Usually 5 to 15 minutes a day is reasonable. Relaxation sound enrichment or mind enrichment techniques can be helpful to use while inverted.

When people first try inversion therapy, they often feel a sensation of being almost upside down even when their head is tilted only slightly below the horizontal position. With regular inversion therapy, people have a more accurate sensation of where their head and body are located. Inversion therapy might help people by reducing stress and improving well-being. Inversion therapy is not appropriate for people with certain medical conditions including heart disease, eye disease, etc. People should always get clearance from their medical doctor or ear specialist before trying inversion therapy. Follow manufacturer recommendations if you are using an inversion table. If you are trying inversion therapy, start out with a very gradual tilt and only increase the tilt slowly as comfortable for you. Any comfortable tilt that places your feet higher than your head is reasonable for ongoing therapy.

Laser Therapy or **Light Therapy** has been used for many years in Europe to treat inner ear difficulties including vertigo (imbalance) and tinnitus. It is often used in combination with gingko biloba (herbal treatment). Low Level Laser Therapy (LLLT) uses light in the visible to near visible (red and near infrared) range of the spectrum. The laser beams are cool to the touch and reportedly do not cause discomfort. They are aimed into the ear canal and through the mastoid bone behind the ear. The idea is that the light or laser irradiation stimulates cells leading to regeneration and healing. Many people with tinnitus report reduced tinnitus pitch and/or volume after treatment. However, some people report worse tinnitus after treatment at least on a temporary basis. While some researchers have suggested this type of treatment can also improve hearing, this has not been confirmed by other studies.

Available studies have used different treatment protocols (e.g. laser positioning, light dosages, length of session, treatment frequency, etc.) or had flaws in how the study was carried out. This has made it difficult to prove any benefit of this therapy. More research is needed to better identify if laser or light therapy treatments are truly effective for tinnitus, and if so which treatment protocols are best. Low Level Laser Therapy (LLLT) should be viewed cautiously until more consistent scientific data is available. If you are considering LLLT, you should get clearance from your medical doctor or ear specialist before starting this type of therapy.

Magnesium deficiency has been linked with tinnitus, sound sensitivity, and increased risk of noise-induced hearing loss. Magnesium is also sometimes called the calming or anti-stress mineral. Food sources of magnesium include nuts, whole grains, legumes and green leafy vegetables. People may want to consider taking a regular daily supplement that contains magnesium to maintain healthy levels in your system. If taking a magnesium supplement, make sure it is in a form that is absorbable by the body. It is not recommended that people take "mega-doses" of any supplement. Supplements should not be taken without clearance from a medical doctor.

Magnetic Treatment using rare earth magnets placed in the ear canal has been suggested as a tinnitus treatment. No benefit has been shown in research studies. Research is still exploring various types of electromagnetic brain stimulation as a tinnitus treatment.

Marijuana has been found helpful to treat some forms of chronic pain or chronic illness. There is currently no published scientific evidence-based research on the use of marijuana to treat tinnitus. Certain people report that marijuana helps with relaxation and stress reduction. There may be negative side effects from smoking marijuana (reduced oxygen flow, skin damage, impaired mental function, etc.). It can be used in other forms (e.g. baked into a recipe such as brownies), although mental function would still be impaired or altered. If you are interested, discuss with your family doctor or ear specialist whether medicinal marijuana would be appropriate to help you cope better with any distress. Medicinal marijuana is not legal in all countries.

Massage can assist with stress reduction especially if received regularly. Massage can help with relaxation in general.

Meditation can assist with stress reduction especially if practiced regularly. Meditation can help with relaxation in general. Depending on the technique used, it can also distract the mind by concentrating attention on specific thoughts or images (e.g. some people concentrate on a candle for this method).

Migraine Treatment is helpful for people with tinnitus and migraine headaches. People who get migraines are more likely to have tinnitus. Tinnitus often becomes louder during a migraine. Treatment for migraines (e.g. prescription medication, chiropractic, cranio-sacral therapy, massage, stress management, etc.) can reduce the frequency and severity of these debilitating headaches. Effective treatment that leads to migraine reduction can help with better tinnitus coping and well-being overall.

Naturopathic Medicine or **Naturopathy** is a professional therapy including diet, exercise and supplements. Therapy focuses on our natural healing abilities and how to enhance them. There is no scientific evidence to show that this type of therapy is effective in general for tinnitus, although it might help certain individuals.

Neuromuscular Dentistry focuses on correcting jaw misalignments or jaw dysfunction (temporomandibular dysfunction or TMD). This type of dentistry focuses on improving position and function of the temporomandibular or jaw joint (TMJ), typically through use of special appliances that guide the jaw and related muscles into a relaxed position. Research suggests that many people with tinnitus and jaw problems report tinnitus improvement after TMD treatment.

Osteopathy is a system of manipulative therapy. Manipulative techniques are used to treat the whole body rather than just the spine. This therapy approach might help with pain reduction and health in general for people with tinnitus and body pain.

Pain Management is an effective treatment tool for tinnitus. There is a higher incidence of tinnitus in people with chronic pain. Any effective treatment for pain (e.g. prescription medication, physiotherapy, chiropractic, massage, stress reduction, tools or devices, etc.) can improve well-being and coping abilities in general.

Positive Thinking has long been a useful approach used by people to cope better with chronic conditions. Positive people try not to focus on negatives, and instead try to focus on what is good in their life. Beethoven had significant hearing loss and "frightful" tinnitus, but carried on writing incredible music up to the end of his life. Famous people with tinnitus include Irish playwright Oscar Wilde, American president Dwight D. Eisenhower, entertainers Barbra Streisand and William Shatner, and musicians like Eric Clapton. They all carried on with their lives and careers regardless of having tinnitus. An Australian man named Nick Vujicic was born with no arms and no legs. He travels around giving speeches to spread the message of living live without limits by focusing on what you *can* do.

Life is what you make of it. Your ears may not be perfect. But if you stop to think about it, you can always find some good things in your life. Hopefully you have a roof over your head, a bed to sleep in, food to eat, people to talk to, and things to do. Don't forget about the positive things you still have and all the things you can still do despite having tinnitus, hearing loss, or sound sensitivity. People who have a positive approach to life cope better with the ups and downs that life throws their way.

Prayer is one of the oldest pain management techniques. Given the similarities between tinnitus and chronic pain, prayer can be helpful to improve coping for some people. The Serenity Prayer is one example: "Grant me the serenity to accept the things I can't change, the courage to change the things I can, and the wisdom to know the difference." Prayer is similar to some relaxation techniques, but can also be helpful as a distraction technique. As with other relaxation approaches, prayer is least effective when used alone and more effective when used in combination with other coping strategies.

Reflexology is a system of therapy where massage or pressure on certain reflex points (usually in the feet) can stimulate and balance energy flow through the body. Although it is unclear how reflexology works, it has been shown to have considerable benefit for pain relief and stress-related conditions. This approach can help by reducing stress and increasing feelings of relaxation.

Reiki is a Japanese technique of stress reduction and relaxation that also promotes healing for various conditions. The technique involves the practitioner placing their hands on or near the body in different positions or near a specific body part in the case of an injury or problem area. Treatments are said to give feelings of relaxation, peace and well-being. A series of treatment may be needed for chronic conditions, or regular treatment may be recommended to maintain well-being. This approach can help with stress relief and relaxation in general.

Self Regulation Therapy (SRT) was developed to relieve uncomfortable or painful emotional and/or physical symptoms including symptoms caused by traumatic events. It is offered through some counselling specialists. Treatment is intended to balance or regulate the nervous system by reducing excess activation. Excess activation comes from accumulated fight or flight response energy that wasn't released when a stressful event occurred. The idea is that humans tend to bottle up their reactions to upsetting, frightening or traumatic experiences instead of experiencing and letting out these natural physical reactions (e.g. try to hold back or hide tears, trembling or physical symptoms when stressed). When left unreleased, the energy from these reactions is stored in the nervous system and can cause various symptoms including anxiety, depression, fatigue, pain, etc. SRT is reported to relieve these symptoms as well as tinnitus and sound sensitivity. Some therapists also offer modified forms of self regulation for stress management.

Sudden onset tinnitus or sound sensitivity can be a stressful event that can also be related to a traumatic event (e.g. head injury, acoustic trauma, etc.). It is unknown whether SRT would be more helpful for sudden onset tinnitus or sound sensitivity than for other types (e.g. gradually developing over time).

Shiatsu therapy is based on Oriental traditional medicine. The treatment approach and philosophy is similar to acupuncture. Instead of needles, pressure is applied to specific body areas to balance energy flow and help healing. This approach can help by improving relaxation and well-being in general.

Spirituality relates to people's interest in the meaning of what it is to be human over and above our physical bodies and material things. Various world religions or spiritually based traditions help people increase their sense of spirituality. Studies are now showing that people with a greater sense of spirituality are better able to manage change and stress, and are better able to recover from sickness or disease.

St. John's Wort is an herb used for tinnitus treatment. It is also used in preparations used to treat mild to moderate depression. Research has not found a beneficial effect in general for tinnitus, although certain individuals might have some benefit. There are some anecdotal or personal reports that this herb can help people with tinnitus. As with other herbal type treatments, St. John's Wort could have side effects or interact with other prescription medications. Any drugs (including this type of herbal treatment) should never be taken without clearance from a medical doctor.

Stress Management strategies or therapies can help people with tinnitus or sound sensitivity cope better, especially those people struggling with anxiety or feeling "stressed out". There are therapists that specialize in stress management treatment. Various books and courses also cover stress management techniques that can be helpful.

Support Groups for tinnitus or sound sensitivity may be available on the Internet or in people's local community. It is natural for people to look for answers from others with the same symptom. Unfortunately, information from some support groups is extremely negative and may only increase feelings of distress. Avoid any negativity like the plague. Any negative sources are not up to date on current treatment methods, since it is well established that there are helpful treatment approaches available. Seek out support groups or people who are working towards coping better and using effective treatments. Getting support from positive people can help make their reality become your reality.

Having support is also helpful to get through flare-ups or rough patches. Often people with chronic conditions like tinnitus or sound sensitivity feel alone because other people just don't understand what it's like. If there are no support groups available, it can be helpful to find support from other people in your day to day contacts who are also dealing with chronic conditions. These people usually have a better understanding of what it is like to deal with something on an ongoing basis whether that is tinnitus, sound sensitivity, pain or some other chronic health condition. Support from an understanding person can help with coping.

Tai Chi or Tai Chi Chuan is a system of gentle physical exercise and stretching. It was developed in China approximately 2000 years ago. It involves a series of postures or movements that flow into each other without pausing. The gentle flowing poses are sometimes called "meditation in motion". Tai Chi is said to improve relaxation, balance and agility, reduce stress, and promote feelings of well-being. This type of exercise can help some people by reducing stress and increasing feelings of relaxation.

Transcranial Magnetic Stimulation is a non-invasive technique that uses strong magnetic fields to stimulate electrical currents in the brain. Research suggests that repetitive Transcranial Magnetic Stimulation (rTMS) is beneficial for various conditions including tinnitus. It is clinically available in some countries.

Ultrasonic Cleaners or scalers are devices used by dental hygienists to help clean teeth. Many people report tinnitus after having their teeth cleaned by these devices. People with tinnitus (or sound sensitivity) may want to ask their dental office not to use this type of device to clean their teeth. Other methods are available (e.g. scaling by hand using dental tools).

Yoga is an ancient practice of exercise developed in India. It is a method to gain power or control over the body and mind. Yoga usually includes physical techniques or postures, breathing techniques, and mental techniques (e.g. meditation). Yoga or exercise studios usually offer various methods of yoga with classes for anyone from beginners to experts. Yoga is often recommended for people with tinnitus. Yoga can reduce stress and increase feelings of relaxation.

Zinc levels may be low in some people with tinnitus. The highest concentration of zinc in our bodies is in the inner ear. Some studies have shown that people with low zinc levels had a decrease in tinnitus after taking zinc supplements. People may want to consider taking a regular daily vitamin and mineral supplement that contains zinc to maintain healthy levels in their bodies. It is not recommended that people with tinnitus take "mega-doses" of any supplement. Any vitamins or minerals for tinnitus should never be taken without clearance from a medical doctor.

> **Author's Case:** I have tried various alternative approaches including acupuncture, amalgam (mercury) filling removal, antioxidants, B vitamins, chiropractic, cranio-sacral therapy, food allergy avoidance, gingko biloba, homeopathy, inversion therapy, magnesium, meditation, migraine treatment, naturopathic medicine, Tai Chi, ultrasonic cleaner avoidance, yoga and zinc.
>
> For me, many of these approaches have helped decrease stress, improve relaxation and increase overall well-being. Gingko biloba reduced overall tinnitus loudness for me up to a point. In my case it would be useful for flare-ups. When I accidentally have foods I am allergic to, my tinnitus definitely flares up. Food allergy avoidance is

important for me. My dental office was unhappy when I asked them not to use the ultrasonic cleaner on my teeth. I switched to a dental office that was comfortable using other methods (e.g. hand scaling). When doing yoga, if I bend over upside down and balance on one leg with my head turned to the left my tinnitus disappears. This pose is not practical to maintain in daily life. Still I enjoy the relaxation and flexibility yoga gives me.

For ongoing health maintenance, I eat a diet high in antioxidants and use chiropractic, food allergy avoidance, occasional inversion therapy and yoga. I also take supplements that contain B vitamins, magnesium and zinc. I also have certain supportive people that I know I can talk to about how I am doing, and this helps me cope better.

Other Cases: The author has clients who have tried various alternative approaches. Individual benefit varies greatly between people. Sometimes approaches help with overall coping and well-being. Sometimes tinnitus benefit is found.

FUTURE HOPE

The future depends on what we do in the present.
Mahatma Ghandi.

The first recorded tinnitus treatments date back to ancient Mesopotamian clay tablets. Ancient treatments included exorcisms to get rid of ghosts in the ear, incantations or prayers whispered into the ears, and herbal treatments. These tablets also show that physicians or care providers at that time reassured people that treatment could help. The ancient Greeks were aware of the effect sound had on tinnitus, and sound has long been used to treat tinnitus. The first formal reference to sound enrichment was in the 1800's. Sound types included music or the sound from a fire. In one case a person even moved to live next to a watermill so they could hear the sound of water as the mill's waterwheel turned. Currently there are many effective treatment approaches available with some similarities and differences to ancient times.

The challenge now with tinnitus is that there is no single treatment that works for all people with distressing tinnitus. With ongoing research, it is hoped that there will be better tinnitus evaluation and better identification of which specific treatment will work best for each individual rather than through the current process of "try and see". As well as better targeting treatment, research is also exploring improvements to current treatments and exploring new treatments. A few promising ideas include better in-ear devices and hearing aids, drug treatment, inner ear stimulation, and maybe even one day inner ear repair.

Current in-ear devices (e.g. in-ear sound generators or combination devices) are very limited in technology features and in the type of sound available. With ongoing advances in technology, there is significant room for improvement. In the future, devices should be able to offer a variety of sound types customized for each individual. This might range from noise focused at specific frequencies to specific sounds that could be much more beneficial for people with tinnitus than what is currently available.

Hearing aid manufacturers are also exploring hearing aids that can play specific sound types. These hearing aids would have advanced digital hearing aid technology along with tailored sound enrichment programs. Research is currently investigating various sounds and music to see which would be most beneficial to have available in hearing aids for people with tinnitus. Researchers are also looking at whether it would be helpful to fit hearing aids on people with tinnitus that have normal hearing as part of a tinnitus treatment program.

New forms of drug treatment are being researched. In the past, certain drugs (e.g. lidocaine) were explored as possible tinnitus treatments. However, often these drugs needed to be administered by injection, caused severe negative side effects, and only gave brief temporary relief. Currently there are certain drugs used to treat various conditions (e.g. alcoholism, epilepsy, Alzheimer's, depression, etc.) that are also found to reduce or eliminate tinnitus. Various researchers are exploring these drugs as potential tinnitus treatment options. The goal is to find the best dose of drugs that can be taken in a pill form and have beneficial long lasting results on tinnitus without negative side effects.

Researchers are also looking at electrical stimulation of the inner ear to reduce tinnitus loudness or intensity. Cochlear implants used for people with profound hearing loss are an example of electrical stimulation since the device itself generates electric signals within the inner ear. Many people with cochlear implants notice reduced tinnitus once the device is working. The cochlear implant surgical procedure is not an option for tinnitus patients unless they have no useable hearing. Research is looking into the possibility of surgical electrical implants for people with tinnitus and better hearing.

Researchers around the world also continue to study how our complex hearing system works, and how the inner ear hearing structures might be repaired. It is interesting that certain species (e.g. birds, frogs and fish) can repair inner ear structures by re-growing them after damage. This allows them to hear again after being deafened. Research is exploring whether mammals like humans might be able to do the same thing. It will be a long time before researchers discover if this is possible and how it can be done. But since tinnitus is often associated with hearing loss, the ability to grow replacement hearing structures could be a large step towards a cure for both hearing loss and tinnitus.

There are always new tinnitus treatments being reported. Tinnitus treatment has come a long way from trying to get rid of ear ghosts. But potential new therapies are not necessarily a well-researched improvement. When you hear about a new treatment, it is best to check with your audiologist, tinnitus specialist or ear specialist. They are able to help review any new research, and determine whether the treatment is available and appropriate for your individual needs. Tinnitus associations in various countries can also be great resources for current information on ongoing tinnitus research.

Harrier Beecher Stowe once said, "when you get into a tight place and everything goes against you, till it seems as though you could not hang on a minute longer, never give up then, for that is just the place and time that the tide will turn." It is now a hopeful time for tinnitus. There has never been so much research on underlying tinnitus mechanisms and tinnitus treatments. There is truly hope that researchers will find a treatment or approach that will cure tinnitus. In the meantime, use the treatment tools available to you to reduce any tinnitus distress. There is tinnitus treatment help available now, and it does work. Use that treatment help and turn the tide. In a 2005 interview with the American Tinnitus Association, the talented entertainer William Shatner talks about how he has severe tinnitus, but it doesn't disrupt his life because he uses coping strategies. Mr. Shatner also points out that in the end, "It is only a noise…It is simply and utterly a noise."

CONCLUSION

Tinnitus is an internally generated noise that distresses some people. Sound sensitivity is a reduced tolerance or distress for sounds that do not bother other people. Current theories suggest that tinnitus and sound sensitivity come from overactive nerve fiber networks in the brain. Treatment tools required are based on how much distress a person has. Choose the specific tools (e.g. sound types, distraction techniques, relaxation techniques, etc.) that speak most directly to your individual needs. Keep track of what works for intensive care, ongoing care and flare-up care.

TINNITUS TREATMENT

1. See your doctor and/or ear specialist (e.g. Otologist or Otolaryngologist) to rule out any medical condition requiring treatment.

2. See an audiologist or tinnitus specialist for a tinnitus evaluation and education and reassurance counselling.

3. If you have hearing loss, get appropriate hearing aid(s). Try communication strategies and/or assistive listening devices.

4. If you have hazardous noise exposure, use appropriate hearing protection.

5. If you still have daytime distress, use distraction sound enrichment and distraction mind enrichment. Some people also benefit from relaxation sound enrichment and relaxation or imagination mind enrichment in the day as needed.

6. If you have nighttime distress, use relaxation sound enrichment. Some people also benefit from relaxation or imagination mind enrichment and sleep management strategies.

7. Consider other options as appropriate for your individual needs such as body enrichment, alternative approaches, etc.

8. For more severe distress, get formal tinnitus therapy or counselling therapy. Formal therapy is usually offered through a tinnitus or counselling specialist. If you have severe distress and will be going to formal tinnitus therapy, it is usually best to get hearing aids or other devices as prescribed by your tinnitus specialist. Medication for sleep or emotional distress may also be needed until you are able to cope better using other treatment tools.

SOUND SENSITIVITY TREATMENT

1. See your doctor and/or ear specialist (e.g. Otologist or Otolaryngologist) to rule out any medical condition requiring treatment.

2. See an audiologist or tinnitus specialist for evaluation and education and reassurance counselling.

3. If your sound sensitivity requires treatment, it should be treated first before tinnitus treatment (if needed).

4. Try not to avoid regular everyday sounds.

5. Use soft day and night relaxation sound enrichment to help de-sensitize your ears. White noise is sometimes used. Pink noise is also known to be helpful for sound sensitivity.

6. Use relaxation mind enrichment as needed. Some people also benefit from other types of mind enrichment (e.g. imagination, distraction, etc.).

7. Do not overprotect your ears. If you are very bothered by loud uncomfortable everyday sounds, try using appropriate hearing protection for daytime use (e.g. filtered earplugs). The goal would be to wean off these as much as possible over time.

8. If you have hazardous noise exposure, use appropriate hearing protection.

9. For more severe distress, get formal sound sensitivity therapy or counselling therapy. Formal sound sensitivity therapy is available through tinnitus specialists. Auditory Retraining Therapy (a modified version of Tinnitus Retraining Therapy used for sound sensitivity) is

available through TRT specialists. Counselling therapy is available through counselling specialists. If you work in hazardous noise, your care provider can guide you on any adjustments you need to make for work while you are going through treatment. Medication for sleep or emotional distress may be needed until you are able to cope better using other treatment tools.

10. Once your sound sensitivity has improved, get tinnitus treatment if needed.

ABOUT THE AUTHOR

J. L. Mayes is a clinical audiologist and "tinnitus coach" with over 20 years of experience. She is a registered member with the British Columbia College of Speech and Hearing Health Professionals. She specializes in workplace noise-induced and trauma related hearing loss and tinnitus, and has a diploma in adult education. She lives and works in the lower mainland of Vancouver, British Columbia, Canada.

The author has also had tinnitus for over 20 years. After being told to "just learn to live with it", she spent years with severe tinnitus and severe tinnitus distress trying to figure out how to live with it. Over the years, she has used various traditional and alternative approaches described throughout this book. The result so far is a mild to moderate tinnitus sound with little distress. It is still there when she listens for it or when it is too quiet around. But her tinnitus is rarely bothersome.

Perhaps one day in the future, a new treatment will come out that can get rid of it completely. Until then, she will keep using all the tools at her disposal to live and cope well. She hopes this book will help other people distressed by tinnitus find treatment tools that will help them cope better without distress in their daily life. For now the goal is improved well-being through coping strategies and treatment. For the future, there is hope for a cure. Stay hopeful as you care for your tinnitus. Onward and upward.

If this book only helps even just one person out there, then the journey has been worth it.

DEFINITIONS

Acclimatization is an improvement in benefit (usually in speech understanding) that happens after a person is fit with hearing aids. It usually takes approximately two to three months to acclimatize to hearing aids.

Acoustic Reflex Testing is a test that uses extremely loud beeps to trigger a very small muscle reflex that pulls on the stirrup (stapes) middle ear bone. This test helps check how well the middle ear system is working. Because very loud test tones are used, it is not recommended for people with tinnitus or sound sensitivity.

Acoustic Trauma refers to the effects of an acute noise hazard from a single or a few exposures to very high levels of sound. Effects can include hearing loss and/or tinnitus. Partial or full recovery can occur depending on the nature of the acoustic trauma.

Acute Noise Hazard may be present for short (e.g. less than 60 seconds) extremely high intensity sound exposure (e.g. gunfire, explosion, etc.). Acute noise hazards can cause acoustic trauma (e.g. hearing loss and/or tinnitus).

Air Conduction is the pathway when sound waves travel through the outer and middle ears to reach the inner ear. Air conduction sound is used during hearing testing to help check how the middle and inner ears work in combination.

Assistive Listening Devices (ALD's) are devices that can be used with hearing aids or alone to help a person hear and understand speech better in difficult or noisy listening situations. Devices may be personal (e.g. FM System) or group (e.g. built into a movie theater or courtroom). Personal or group systems allow speech to be sent directly through a special headset or through a person's hearing aids (if compatible) so that the speech is heard better over background noise.

Attenuation is sound reduction or softening. Attenuation usually refers to the amount sound input is lowered (made quieter) when using hearing protection. People with tinnitus or sound sensitivity should select hearing protection with appropriate attenuation to avoid overprotection.

Audiologists are professionals with specialized education and training in evaluation and non-medical treatment for ear problems including hearing loss and tinnitus.

Audiometer is a machine used to test hearing.

Auditory Brainstem Response (ABR) testing is a specialized hearing system test that uses loud sound to check sound processing along the auditory or hearing nerve.

Auditory Deprivation can happen when people who have fairly equal hearing loss in both ears don't wear two hearing aids. Over time they may gradually lose their ability to understand what people are saying in the unaided ear. Auditory deprivation is the term used to describe the poorer speech understanding in the unaided ear.

Auditory Retraining Therapy is a term sometimes used to describe a modified form of Tinnitus Retraining Therapy (TRT) used to treat sound sensitivity or hyperacusis.

Binaural refers to both ears of an individual.

Body Enrichment is the use of exercise, diet and a healthy lifestyle to help improve coping ability and reduce distress.

Bone Conduction is the pathway when sound waves travel through the bones of the skull to reach the inner ear. Bone conduction sound is used during hearing testing to help check how the inner ear is working.

Chronic Noise Hazard can happen when intense sound exposure (usually 85 dBA or greater) is repeated regularly over time. Chronic noise hazards can cause noise or music-induced hearing loss.

Cognitive Behaviour Therapy (CBT) or Cognitive Behavioural Therapy is a counselling therapy often used to help people with tinnitus distress although it can also be used for sound sensitivity. It is offered through counselling specialists (e.g. psychologists or psychiatrists who are experienced in this approach) and involves learning four main techniques. These include cognitive, distraction, relaxation and imagination techniques.

Cognitive Technique is a therapy technique that helps people reduce or eliminate negative or unhelpful thoughts. It is usually used as part of Cognitive Behaviour Therapy (CBT). Counselling specialists can teach people these techniques that help improve coping and reduce distress.

Combination Device is a sound enrichment or sound therapy device that combines a hearing aid and in-ear sound generator. Combination devices may be recommended for people with hearing loss and severe tinnitus distress or sound sensitivity.

Communication Systems include cell phones, digital wireless phones, or other communication system technology. Various hearing aid manufacturers now offer products with communication system compatibility.

Complete Masking is a sound loudness used to treat tinnitus. Complete masking happens when an outside sound is made loud enough so that the tinnitus can no longer be heard. Many people have tinnitus that can't be completely masked.

Conductive refers to hearing loss caused by problems in the outer or middle ear pathways.

Counselling Specialists are professionals (e.g. counsellors, psychologists, psychiatrists) with specialized training in counselling therapy. Counselling therapy can help improve coping and lower distress.

Counselling Therapy is described under Mind Enrichment.

Decibel (dB) is a unit of measurement for sound intensity. Sound intensity hazardous to human ears is usually measured in dBA.

Dental Appliances fit over the teeth, and are worn in the mouth while sleeping. People with tinnitus use them for various reasons (e.g. stop teeth grinding, reduce jaw pain, treat sleep disorders, etc.). Dental appliances are custom fit to each individual person by a dentist or dental specialist.

Direct Audio Input (DAI) is a hearing aid option that allows a hearing aid to be directly connected to an external audio source such as a television, telephone, computer, CD player, or most commonly an assistive listening device such as an FM System. Hearing aid technology is also available that offers wireless connection depending on the manufacturer.

Directive Counselling is a specific type of counselling therapy used in Tinnitus Retraining Therapy (TRT).

Distraction Sound is a type of sound used for sound enrichment or sound therapy that people can listen to instead of their tinnitus.

Distraction Technique is a technique or therapy that helps people specifically think about other things instead of their tinnitus.

Double-up is when people wear earplugs and earmuffs together to protect their ears from noise or sound around them. Double-up should only be used for extreme noise hazards. Otherwise it can lead to overprotection, which can make tinnitus or sound sensitivity worse.

Eardrum Testing or tympanometry measures the movement and position of the eardrum. This test helps check how well the middle ear system is working.

Early Warning Tinnitus is the tinnitus people sometimes notice after they are exposed to a chronic noise hazard. This is usually a temporary tinnitus that recovers after time away from noise. It is called early warning tinnitus because it is an early warning sign that repeated exposure without hearing protection could lead to permanent hearing loss or tinnitus.

Ear Specialists (e.g. Otologists or Otolaryngologists) are doctors who specialize in evaluating and treating any medical problems related to the ears, hearing or balance systems. It is recommended that people with tinnitus or sound sensitivity see an ear specialist before starting any non-medical treatment.

Electronystagmography (ENG) is a specialized balance system test. It is often used when people have imbalance or dizziness. ENG testing involves sending water into the ears, and it can be loud.

FM Systems are a type of assistive listening device used to help improve speech understanding in background noise. FM Systems use a microphone (e.g. pointed toward the driver in a car, placed in the center of a dinner or conference table, clipped on a shirt collar near the mouth of an instructor, etc.). The voice signal from the microphone is then sent directly to a receiver at a hearing aid or headset. Any surrounding or background noise is minimized. FM systems can be very helpful in various work, school and social situations. Hearing aids must be FM compatible to work with FM Systems.

Fractal Music is a special type of relaxing background music created using a mathematical algorithm or calculation. Listening to fractal music may be beneficial since this type of music is known to lower stress and improve relaxation.

Frequency of a sound depends on how many sound waves reach the ear in a given period of time. The faster the sound waves are moving, the higher the perceived pitch or frequency. Frequency is measured in Hertz (Hz).

Habituation is a term used in Tinnitus Retraining Therapy (TRT). Habituation has happened when a person is no longer aware of their tinnitus except when they focus their attention on it, and even then the tinnitus is not annoying or bothersome.

Hawthorne Effect is when people experience a sense of relief just because someone is doing something for their condition.

Hearing Aids are devices that help people with hearing loss hear better. Hearing aids analyze and process sound as needed for a person's hearing loss. Hearing aids are helpful for people with hearing loss and tinnitus since they improve hearing and give sound enrichment.

Hearing Loss is a reduced ability to hear sounds or voices. Hearing loss usually happens from problems with the outer, middle and/or inner ear. Hearing can be reduced for low, mid and/or high frequency sounds. Severity is usually described by degree from mild to profound. There are many causes of hearing loss.

Hearing Loss Management is the use of appropriate hearing aids to treat hearing loss and tinnitus.

Hearing Protection are devices designed to lower the loudness of hazardous environmental sound to non-hazardous levels by blocking the ear canal or covering up the ear. Hearing protection is available in various earplug and earmuff styles. Hearing protection is also available with various amounts and patterns of sound reduction. People should select a pattern and amount of hearing protection appropriate for hearing loss, tinnitus and/or sound sensitivity.

Hearing Protection Management is the use of appropriate hearing protection for people with hearing loss, tinnitus and/or sound sensitivity.

Hertz (Hz) is the unit of measurement for sound frequency.

Hyperacusis is described under Sound Sensitivity.

Idiopathic means the cause is unknown. Tinnitus and hearing loss are often idiopathic.

Imagination Technique is a technique or therapy (formally called guided imagery) that helps people use their imagination to calm their thoughts by using mental pictures or images.

In-Ear Sound Generator is a sound enrichment or sound therapy device that may be recommended to treat severe tinnitus distress or sound sensitivity. These devices are worn on the ears, and usually make a white noise sound.

Inner Ear is the anatomical section of the ear made up of a small snail shaped structure called the cochlea. The cochlea is a complex fluid filled structure that responds to incoming sound and changes the sound vibrations into electrical impulses. Technically the inner ear includes structures for hearing (cochlea) and for balance.

Intensity of a sound depends on how large the sound waves are that reach the ear. The larger the sound wave is, the louder or more intense the perceived sound. Intensity is measured in decibels (dB).

Loudness is a subjective perception of sound intensity (e.g. soft or loud).

Loudness Discomfort Level (LDL) testing is used to check a person's loudness comfort range. LDL's are checked across a frequency range to identify when sounds become uncomfortable. If LDL's are lower than normal (e.g. loudness would not be ok for regular everyday sound intensities), then a person may have sound sensitivity.

Loudness Match is a match of a person's tinnitus loudness to the intensity (measured in decibel or dB) of a sound sent through an audiometer. The loudness match is usually measured at a person's tinnitus pitch match. Loudness matches tend to be fairly stable over time. Note the sone is actually the unit used for loudness measurement. The dB to sone conversion is not usually calculated in clinical practice. Measurements in dB can underestimate perceived loudness.

Loudness Recruitment is a rapid growth in the perception of loudness often seen with sensorineural or inner ear hearing loss. Even though a person has hearing loss, loud sounds (above hearing thresholds) still seem loud similar to how they would for a person with normal hearing.

Masking is a term sometimes used to describe the effect of sound loudness on tinnitus. Sound loudness may be set to non-masking, partial masking, mixing or complete masking to treat tinnitus depending on the treatment approach being used.

Middle Ear is the anatomical section of the ear that includes the eardrum and middle ear bones that sit in an air filled space between the eardrum and the inner ear.

Mind Enrichment is a tinnitus or sound sensitivity treatment approach that may include various mind techniques or counselling therapy. Formal counselling therapy is usually offered by counselling specialists although some counselling therapy is offered by tinnitus specialists. Mind enrichment is often most helpful in combination with sound enrichment or sound therapy.

Minimum Masking Level (MML) is a test sometimes used to measure the effect of sound on tinnitus. The MML is the softest level of noise that makes a person unable to hear their tinnitus.

Mixed refers to a hearing loss with both a sensorineural and conductive component.

Mixing is a sound loudness used to treat tinnitus. This term is specific to Tinnitus Retraining Therapy (TRT). Mixing is when an outside sound is turned to a loudness where it begins to mix or blend with the tinnitus but does not change or cover up the tinnitus sound.

Monaural refers to one ear of an individual.

Multiple Microphones are a directional sound capability option on many current hearing aids. Multiple microphones work together to reduce sounds coming from behind you so that the sound or voice you are facing is amplified or increased. This feature makes it easier to hear conversations when in background noise.

Music-Induced Hearing Loss is a permanent high frequency hearing loss from repeated exposure to intense music over time. The loss is similar to the noise-induced hearing loss caused by any chronic noise hazard.

Noise is often defined as an unwanted or unpleasant sound.

Noise Hazard is described under Acute Noise Hazard and Chronic Noise Hazard.

Noise-Induced Hearing Loss is a permanent hearing loss that can develop from chronic or acute noise hazards. Chronic noise hazards typically cause a pattern of high pitch hearing loss in both ears. There can be temporary hearing shift and early warning tinnitus that appears first. With repeated unprotected exposure, permanent noise-induced hearing loss and tinnitus can develop. Acute noise hazards may cause hearing loss in one ear or worse in one ear depending on which ear is closest to the intense sound event. The hearing loss or tinnitus from acute noise hazards can be temporary or permanent with partial to full recovery possible if there is no repeated unprotected exposure.

Noise Reduction Processing is a feature offered in many hearing aids that usually helps improve sound quality or listening comfort. Some forms of noise reduction are designed to screen out soft environmental sounds and any internal noise created by the hearing aid's own microphones. This type of noise reduction is not necessarily helpful for people with tinnitus when they are in quiet environments.

Noise Reduction Rating (NRR) indicates how much sound reduction (in dB) specific hearing protection (earmuff or earplug) will provide. The NRR is usually marked on the packaging. Wearing hearing protection with NRR that is too high for the surrounding noise environment can lead to overprotection.

Non-Masking is a sound loudness used to treat tinnitus. Non-masking happens when an outside sound is turned to a loudness where it can be heard, but it does not blend together with or cover up the tinnitus sound.

Occlusion is when the ear canals are closed or blocked off.

Occlusion Effect can happen if hearing aids are a style that causes occlusion by blocking off a person's ear canals. With hearing aid occlusion, natural sound seems muffled, a person's voice can sound strange or loud, and tinnitus can seem louder. People with tinnitus should use hearing aid styles that occlude or block off their ears as little as possible.

Open Fitting is a hearing aid style that reduces or eliminates the occlusion effect.

Otoacoustic Emissions Test measures emissions or responses from the inner ear. Testing is done across a range of frequencies. This test mainly helps check the status of the inner ear, although middle ear problems can affect whether emissions are present or absent.

Otoscope is a device that provides specialized lighting for a visual check of the ear canal and eardrum.

Outer Ear is the anatomical section of the ear that includes the visible part of the ear (pinna) and ear canal.

Overprotection is when the hearing protection being used gives too much sound reduction for the person's noise exposure. Overprotection is very undesirable for people with tinnitus and/or sound sensitivity since it can make both conditions worse. Overprotection is also a problem for people with hearing loss since it can make it harder to hear necessary sounds or voices while using hearing protection. People with hearing loss, tinnitus and/or sound sensitivity should select appropriate hearing protection to avoid overprotection.

Partial Masking is a sound loudness used to treat tinnitus. Partial masking is when an outside sound is turned to a loudness where it begins to mix or blend with the tinnitus sound.

Pink Noise contains sound with more energy at lower frequencies. It is similar to the range of everyday sound, and may be helpful to treat sound sensitivity.

Pinna is the visible part of the ear commonly used to hang glasses or earrings on.

Pitch is a subjective perception of sound frequency (e.g. low or high tone).

Pitch Match is a match of the person's tinnitus pitch to the frequency (Hertz) of a sound sent through the audiometer. Pitch matches tend to be variable over time.

Progressive Tinnitus Management (PTM) is a tinnitus treatment approach used by audiologists. It includes counselling and sound enrichment or sound therapy as needed by each individual person. The sound therapy uses various sound types and sound devices with sound loudness set to whatever is most helpful (e.g. non-masking, partial masking or complete masking). Psychologists may also assist by providing Cognitive Behaviour Therapy. PTM guidance on how to manage may be offered one-on-one or in group education sessions.

Pulsed Tones are a series of short pulsed tones used during hearing testing (e.g. bip bip bip). Pulsed tones are recommended during hearing testing for people with tinnitus to make it easier for them to distinguish the test tones from their tinnitus.

Real Ear Measurement is a test done with a hearing aid working in the ear. Real ear measurement checks how well a hearing aid is amplifying or increasing sound for the wearer's hearing loss.

Relaxation Sound is calm or relaxing sound used for sound enrichment or sound therapy.

Relaxation Technique is a technique or therapy that helps people feel calm or relaxed.

Residual Inhibition (RI) refers to the effect when tinnitus perception can be reduced in loudness or eliminated completely after sound is presented to the ear. For most people, RI effects are usually very short and only last at most a few seconds or minutes after the sound is turned off.

Sensorineural refers to hearing loss from problems in the inner ear or along the auditory or hearing nerve.

Severity Ranking Scales are informal scales used to rank tinnitus or tinnitus distress severity. For example, how bothersome is it on a scale of 1 to 100? Formal tinnitus questionnaires are often used instead of ranking scales.

Sleep Disorders (e.g. snoring, sleep apnea) can affect how a person breathes while they are asleep. Sleep may be disturbed if a person with tinnitus or their sleep partner has a sleep disorder. Sleep disorders can be evaluated by a sleep specialist or sleep clinic.

Sone is the unit of measurement used in loudness scales. A calculation is needed to convert intensity (dB) into the sone. This is not routinely done in actual clinical practice. A tinnitus loudness match is usually measured in dB. This can underestimate perceived loudness.

Sound Devices are devices used for sound enrichment or sound therapy. A large variety of devices can be used from tabletop to worn in the ears. Different sound types can be played through devices depending on what is needed.

Sound Enrichment or sound therapy is the specific use of sound to treat tinnitus or sound sensitivity. Various sound types and sound devices are used for day and/or night sound enrichment. Treatment and devices are usually available through audiologists or tinnitus specialists. Sound enrichment is most often effective in combination with mind enrichment or counselling therapy.

Sound Pillow is a pillow with a built-in speaker for playing sound. When using a sound pillow, only the person with their head on the pillow can hear the sound. Some people make their own sound pillow by using a flat speaker (e.g. from an audio equipment store) placed inside their regular pillow. Sound pillows can be used with tabletop sound machines for sound enrichment or sound therapy while sleeping.

Sound Sensitivity refers to discomfort or pain from ordinary everyday sounds that are not loud or distressing to other people. The condition is a reduced tolerance to sound that can range from mild to very severe. Sound sensitivity may be referred to by various terms including hyperacusis, phonophobia, misophonia, etc. Sound sensitivity is reversible with treatment. It is usually treated before tinnitus distress if a person has both. Treatment usually includes sound therapy (sound enrichment), counselling therapy (mind enrichment) and hearing protection management. Tinnitus specialists and/or counselling specialists usually offer treatment for sound sensitivity.

Sound Therapy is described under Sound Enrichment.

Sound Types are various sounds used for sound enrichment or sound therapy. Sound types can include music, white noise or other distraction or relaxation sound.

Tabletop Sound Machine is a sound generating device that sits on a table in a room or at a person's bedside. These devices usually have a variety of sound types (e.g. white noise, rain, etc.). They are used for sound enrichment or sound therapy to help people add sound into their environment. They are often recommended for quiet activities or sleeping. Some tabletop sound machines are compatible with pillow speakers so only the person with their head on the pillow can hear the sound while sleeping.

Telecoil or t-coil is an option that allows a hearing aid to pick up the electromagnetic voice signal coming through a telephone, and then amplify it through the hearing aid. Some assistive listening devices also work through telecoils. Newer hearing aid technology on the market also offers other forms of telephone and communication system compatibility depending on the manufacturer.

Temporary Hearing Shift or temporary threshold shift is a short term hearing change (muffled or impaired hearing) after unprotected exposure to hazardous noise. This temporary hearing change gradually recovers over time. If there is repeated exposure without hearing protection, then permanent hearing loss can develop. Temporary hearing shift often happens along with early warning tinnitus.

Threshold is defined as the softest intensity (loudness) a person can hear a specific sound (e.g. tone or word).

Tinnitus is a name given to noises in the ears that are heard when there is no outside noise source. Tinnitus is commonly pronounced [tin-it-us] or [tin-night-us]. Tinnitus can be described as ringing, roaring, hissing, screeching, whistling, clicking, humming, buzzing, chirping, pounding, pulsing or combinations of sound effects. It is very common. Many people with tinnitus are not distressed or bothered by it.

Tinnitus Distress refers to the variety of emotions experienced by some people in response to their tinnitus. Emotions may include anxiety, fear, annoyance, irritability, anger, sadness, depression, etc. There are various effective treatments or therapies available for people who have tinnitus distress. Audiologists, tinnitus specialists and/or counselling specialists usually offer treatment.

Tinnitus Evaluation is a detailed evaluation for people with tinnitus that usually includes an interview, hearing assessment, tinnitus assessment, sound sensitivity assessment (if necessary), tinnitus questionnaires, and counselling on results. Audiologists or tinnitus specialists usually do tinnitus evaluations.

Tinnitus Masking Therapy is a specific form of tinnitus sound enrichment or sound therapy that uses partial or complete masking sound. The sound is used at a loudness where the tinnitus is either changed or covered up by the outside sound. Tinnitus masking therapy is usually available through audiologists or tinnitus specialists.

Tinnitus Music Therapy is a specific approach that uses specially processed music to treat tinnitus (e.g. Neuromonics Tinnitus Treatment). It is usually available through an audiologist or tinnitus specialist.

Tinnitus Questionnaires contain standardized lists of questions. The questions are designed to identify problem areas that may be present if a person has tinnitus distress. Tinnitus questionnaires are commonly used as part of a tinnitus evaluation.

Tinnitus Retraining Therapy (TRT) is a specific form of tinnitus treatment that includes directive counselling and sound therapy. The sound therapy is used at a mixing loudness where the tinnitus mixes or blends with the outside sound but is not changed or covered up by it. A modified form of TRT sometimes called Auditory Retraining Therapy may be used to treat sound sensitivity. TRT is usually available through tinnitus specialists.

Tinnitus Specialists are professionals (often audiologists) with specialized training in specific types of tinnitus and sound sensitivity treatment.

Transient Spontaneous Tinnitus (TST) is a short usually high pitch tinnitus lasting a few seconds. Almost everyone hears it occasionally.

White Noise is sound made up of all frequencies, with equal sound energy at each frequency. It sounds like a "shhhhh" type sound. Sound enrichment or sound therapy often uses white noise sound to treat tinnitus or sound sensitivity.

RESOURCES

The resources listed here are only the tip of the iceberg. Keep on the lookout, and check for other positive or helpful associations, organizations, books, Websites and other resources through your care providers, Internet searches and through retailers, libraries or other sources. Tinnitus Association Websites have useful information and resources for people with tinnitus or sound sensitivity (hyperacusis) as well as links to other helpful Websites and resources.

TINNITUS ASSOCIATIONS

Tinnitus Association of Canada
c/o 23 Ellis Park Road
Toronto, ON M6S 2V4
www.kadis.com/ta/tinnitus

American Tinnitus Association
P.O. Box 5
Portland, OR 97207-0005
www.ata.org

Australian Tinnitus Association
P.O. Box 660
Woollahra NSW 1350
Australia
www.tinnitus.asn.au

J. L. Mayes

British Tinnitus Association
Ground Floor, Unit 5
Acorn Business Park, Woodseats Close
Sheffield S8 0TB
www.tinnitus.org.uk

European Federation of Tinnitus Associations
www.eutinnitus.com

SOUND MACHINES AND CDS

Various retail stores or Websites sell CDs, devices, or tabletop machines that play various sounds or sound effects. As a starting point, try Websites such as www.sound-oasis.com, www.healthjourneys.com or www.liquidmindmusic.com. Also search or check product catalogues under key words like white noise, white noise machine, white noise CD, nature sound, nature sound machine, nature sound CD, sleep machine, relaxing sound CD, pink noise, pink noise machine, pink noise CD, etc. If selecting a tabletop sound machine, it should have an auxiliary jack and three main features: a variety of sounds including white noise (and/or pink noise capability if needed for sound sensitivity), a volume control, and no automatic shut-off (after being turned on, the machine should be able to run constantly until turned off). Some people also like battery back up on their sound machine for sleep so it keeps running even if the power goes off.

TINNITUS CDS

Petroff Dynamic Tinnitus Mitigation System™
Petroff Audio Technologies
2278 Keswick Lane
Rock Hill, SC 29732
This therapeutic CD system with noise, nature and relaxation sounds is available through various Websites including www.contactassist.com. That Website also offers other hearing related products.

Moses-Lang Tinnitus CD
OHSU Tinnitus Clinic NRC04
Oregon Health Sciences University
3181 S.W. Sam Jackson Park Road

Portland, OR 97239-3098
www.ohsu.edu/ohrc/tinnitus clinic
CD tracks include white noise and pink noise.

HEARING PROTECTION

Custom-molded earplugs
These are usually available through local audiologists or hearing clinics. For information on Musician's™ earplugs, see www.etymotic.com.

Pre-molded earplugs, banded earplugs or earmuffs
Safety-supply companies are a good place to buy hearing protection equipment. Some retail stores and Websites also offer certain appropriate products as described in the chapter on Hearing Protection Management.

Hearing protection for musicians or music lovers
www.musiciansclinics.com
www.hearnet.com
www.etymotic.com

MRI-safe hearing protection
Hearing protection must be completely non-metallic (not metal detectable). Foam earplugs, reusable silicone earplugs, or non-metallic earmuffs are possible options. Some hospitals or test centres have this hearing protection available for people to use during MRI testing. Various stores and Websites also offer these products.

TINNITUS OR SOUND SENSITIVITY TREATMENT

Cognitive Behaviour(al) Therapy
Various Websites describe counselling approaches including CBT (e.g. www.hopefortinnitus.com).

Hyperacusis Specific Treatment
Various Websites have helpful information including www.hyperacusisnetwork.com and www.hyperacusis.org.

Neuromonics or Music Therapy
www.neuromonics.com

J. L. Mayes

Progressive Tinnitus Management
Various websites describe this approach. The *How To Manage Your Tinnitus* workbook for individuals or *Progressive Tinnitus Management* Bundle for audiologists or care providers are available at www.pluralpublishing.com. The workbook, with store discount for members, is also available at www.ata.org.

Tinnitus Masking Therapy
Various Websites describe this approach.

Tinnitus or Auditory Retraining Therapy
www.tinnitus.org
www.tinnitus-pjj.com

HEARING LOSS MANAGEMENT

Canadian Hearing Society
www.chs.ca

Better Hearing Institute (American)
www.betterhearing.org

British Association for the Hard of Hearing
www.hearingconcern.org/uk

European Federation of Hard of Hearing People (EFHOH)
www.efhoh.org

Self Help for Hard of Hearing People (Australia)
www.shhhaust.org

OTHER WEBSITES

Information on sleep strategies
www.worldsleepfoundation.com
www.sleepfoundation.org

Information on alternative tinnitus treatments or supplements
Available on various Websites including www.tinnitusformula.com.

Try to find information from sites that are based on credible scientific research. Try to avoid sites that contain negative information or that suggest their products will cure everybody.

Information on home-based auditory training program (LACE)

www.neurotone.com

This is a home-based self-paced program used to help train the auditory or hearing system to improve listening and communication skills (e.g. for fast talkers, for speech in background noise, etc.). It was designed for people with hearing loss or listening difficulties. Other sources may also offer auditory training programs for people with hearing problems.

BIBLIOGRAPHY

Since the author was diagnosed with tinnitus in 1986, she has read everything she could find on tinnitus and tinnitus treatment. In the years she spent writing this book, she also read many research studies, books, and articles by various authors on tinnitus and related subjects. The following list includes some of the key references that were reviewed. This list represents the work of many dedicated and expert tinnitus and tinnitus treatment researchers and clinicians. In an early draft of this book, all these articles and books were referenced within the text. However, every reviewer from audiologists to construction workers said the references bogged down the text and made it hard to read. Instead all the main references have been listed in this bibliography. These references have helped form the author's understanding of tinnitus and of current traditional and alternative tinnitus treatments. Any errors or omissions are the author's.

1. Arda, H., Tuncel., U., Akdogan, O., & Ozluoglu, L. (2003) The role of zinc in the treatment of tinnitus. *Otology and Neurotology, 24(1)*, 86–89.

2. Baracca, G., Forti, S., Crocetti, A., Fagnani, E., Scotti, A., Del Bo, L., & Ambrosetti, U. (2007). Results of TRT after eighteen months: Our experience. *International Journal of Audiology, 46*, 217–222.

3. Berger, E. H., Royster, L. H., Royster, J. D., Driscoll, D. P., & Layne, M. (Eds.). (2003). *The Noise Manual*, Revised Fifth Edition. Fairfax, VA: American Industrial Hygiene Association.

4. Cousins, N. (2001). *Anatomy of an Illness as Perceived by the Patient: Reflections on Healing and Regeneration*, Revised Second Edition. W. H. Norton & Company.

5. Davis, P., Paki, B., & Hanley, P. (2007). Neuromonics Tinnitus Treatment: Third Clinical Trial. *Ear and Hearing, 28(2)*, 242–259.

6. Dobie, R. (2003). Depression and tinnitus. *Otolaryngologic Clinics of North America, 36*, 383–388.

7. Evans, M. (1996). The Guide to Natural Therapies: Choosing and Using Natural Methods for Physical and Mental Well-Being. London: Anness Publishing Limited.

8. Folmer, R. L. (2001). Managing chronic tinnitus as phantom auditory pain. *Audiology Online*. www.audiologyonline.com. Retrieved October 15, 2002.

9. Folmer, R. L. (2002). Long-term reductions in tinnitus severity. *BMC Ear, Nose and Throat Disorders, 2*, 3.

10. Folmer, R. L. (2006). Ringing in the ears: Hope and help for tinnitus sufferers. *Deafness Research Foundation*. www.drf.org. Retrieved March 25, 2008.

11. Groves, A. (2008). Can we regenerate the inner ear by teaching old cells new tricks? *Tinnitus Today, 33*, 11–16.

12. Harris, A. (2008). Neuromuscular dentistry – a hopeful path to alignment and tinnitus relief. *Tinnitus Today, 33*, 8–9.

13. Hazell, J. (1999). The TRT method in practice. In J. Hazell (Ed.), *Proceedings of the Sixth International Tinnitus Seminar 1999* (pp. 92–98). London: The Tinnitus and Hyperacusis Centre.

14. Hazell, J., Wood, S., Cooper, H., Stephens, S., Corcoran, A., Coles, R., Baskill, J., & Sheldrake, J. (1985). A clinical study of tinnitus maskers. *British Journal of Audiology, 19*, 65–146.

15. Heller, M. F., & Bergman, M. (1953). Tinnitus in normally hearing persons. *Ann. Otol. 62*, 73–83.

16. Henry, J. A., Jastreboff, M., Jastreboff, P., Schechter, M., & Fausti, S. (2003). Guide to conducting tinnitus retraining therapy initial and follow-up interviews. *Journal of Rehabilitation Research and Development, 40(2)*, 157–178.

17. Henry, J. A., Rheinsburg, B., & Zaugg, T. (2004). Comparison of custom sounds for achieving tinnitus relief. *Journal of the American Academy of Audiology, 15*, 585–598.

18. Henry, J. A., Schechter, M., Nagler, S., & Fausti, S., (2002). Comparison of tinnitus masking and tinnitus retraining therapy. *Journal of the American Academy of Audiology, 13,* 559–581.

19. Henry, J. A., Zaugg, T. L., & Schechter, M. A. (June 2005a). Clinical guide for audiologic tinnitus management I: Assessment. *American Journal of Audiology, 14,* 21–48.

20. Henry, J. A., Zaugg, T. L., & Schechter, M. A. (June 2005b). Clinical guide for audiologic tinnitus management II: Treatment. *American Journal of Audiology, 14,* 49–70.

21. Henry, J. L., & Wilson, P. H. (2001). *The Psychological Management of Chronic Tinnitus: a Cognitive-Behavioural Approach.* Needham Heights, MA: Allyn and Bacon.

22. Henry, J., A., Jastreboff, M., Jastreboff, P., Schechter, M., & Fausti, S. (2002). Assessment of patients for treatment with tinnitus retraining therapy. *Journal of the American Academy of Audiology, 13,* 523–544.

23. Jastreboff, P. J. (1998). Tinnitus: The Method of Pawel J. Jastreboff. In G.A. Gates (ed.). *Current Therapy in Otolaryngology Head and Neck Surgery.* St. Louis: Mosby.

24. Jastreboff, P. J., & Jastreboff, M. M. (2001). Tinnitus retraining therapy. *Seminars in Hearing, 22,* 51–63.

25. Levey, J. & Levey, M. (2003). *The Fine Arts of Relaxation, Concentration, and Meditation.* Boston: Wisdom Publications.

26. Lockwood, A., Salvi, R., & Burkard, R. (2002). Tinnitus. *New England Journal of Medicine, 347(12),* 904–910.

27. Lopez-Gonzalez, M., & Lopez-Fernandez, R., (2004). Sequential sound therapy in tinnitus. *International Tinnitus Journal, 10(2),* 150–55.

28. May, D. & Wray, R. (2005). I've been there: an interview with William Shatner. *Tinnitus Today, 30,* 16–17.

29. McCombe, A., Baguley, D., Coles, R., McKenna, L., McKinney, C., & Windle-Taylor, P. (2001). Guidelines for the grading of tinnitus severity: the results of a working group commissioned by the British Association of Otolaryngologists, Head and Neck Surgeons, 1999. *Clinical Otolaryngology, 26,* 388–393.

30. McFerran, D. & Baguley, D. (2008). The efficacy of treatments for depression used in the management of tinnitus. *Audiological Medicine, 6*, 40–47.

31. McFerran, D., & Phillips, J. (2007). Tinnitus. *The Journal of Laryngology & Otology, 121*, 201–208.

32. McKenna, L. & Irwin, R. (2008). Sound therapy for tinnitus – sacred cow or idol worship?: An investigation of the evidence. *Audiological Medicine, 6*, 16–24.

33. Mohr, A. (2008). Reflections on tinnitus by an existential psychologist. *Audiological Medicine, 6*, 73–77.

34. Moore, T. (1992. *Care of the Soul: A Guide for Cultivating Depth and Sacredness in Everyday Life*. HarperCollins Publishers: New York.

35. Mueller, H. & Hall, J. (1998). *Audiologists' Desk Reference: Audiologic Management, Rehabilitation and Terminology*. San Diego: Singular Publishing Group.

36. Noble, W. & Tyler, R. (2007). Physiology and phenomenology of tinnitus: Implications for treatment. *International Journal of Audiology, 46*, 569–574.

37. Norena, A. J., & Eggermont, J. J. (2005). Enriched acoustic environment after noise trauma reduces hearing loss and prevents cortical map reorganization. *Journal of Neuroscience, 19, 25(3)*, 699–705.

38. Paul, R., & Dennis, K. (1996). What about tinnitus? *American Journal of Audiology, 5*, 5-8.

39. Robinson, S., (2005). Cognitive behaviour therapy—The basics. *Tinnitus Today, 30*, 11–12.

40. Rothwell, J. & Boyd, P. (2008). Amalgam dental fillings and hearing loss. *International Journal of Audiology, 47*, 770–776.

41. Sanders, B. (2002). Noise—its effect on tinnitus. *Tinnitus Today, 27*, 20–30.

42. Scurlock, J., & Stephens, D. (2008). A ringing endorsement for Assyro-Babylonian medicine: The diagnosis and treatment of tinnitus in 1st Millenium BCE Mesopotamia. *Audiological Medicine, 6*, 4–15.

43. Searchfield, G. (2005). Modern hearing aids—a help for tinnitus. *Tinnitus Today, 30,* 14–16.

44. Sindhusake, D., Mitchell, P., Newall, P., Golding, M., Rochtchina, E., & Rubin, G. (2003). Prevalence and characteristics of tinnitus in older adults: the Blue Mountains Hearing Study. *International Journal of Audiology, 42,* 289–294.

45. Sweetow, R. (2001). Hearing aids and tinnitus. *Tinnitus Today, 26,* 14–15.

46. Tyler, R., & Cacae, A. T. (2004). Advances in understanding and treating tinnitus. *Tinnitus Today, 29,* 12–13.

47. Tyler, R., Chang, S., Gehringer, A., & Gogel, S. (2008) Tinnitus: How you can help yourself! *Audiological Medicine, 6(1),* 85–91.

48. Vernon, J. A. (Ed.). (1998). *Tinnitus Treatment and Relief.* Needham Heights, MA: Allyn and Bacon.

49. Wade, P. (2007, Fall). Tinnitus and sleep-disordered breathing. Canadian Hearing Society, *Vibes,* 43–44.

50. Zachriat, C., & Kroner-Herwig, B. (2004). Treating chronic tinnitus: comparison of cognitive-behavioural and habituation-based treatments. *Cognitive Behavioural Therapy, 4, 33(4),* 187–98.